# Management of Bulls

*Editors*

ARTHUR LEE JONES
JOSEPH C. DALTON

## VETERINARY CLINICS
## OF NORTH AMERICA:
## FOOD ANIMAL PRACTICE

www.vetfood.theclinics.com

*Consulting Editor*
ROBERT A. SMITH

March 2024 • Volume 40 • Number 1

**ELSEVIER**

1600 John F. Kennedy Boulevard • Suite 1800 • Philadelphia, Pennsylvania, 19103-2899

http://www.vetfood.theclinics.com

**VETERINARY CLINICS OF NORTH AMERICA: FOOD ANIMAL PRACTICE Volume 40, Number 1**
**March 2024 ISSN 0749-0720, ISBN-13: 978-0-443-13021-2**

Editor: Taylor Hayes
Developmental Editor: Varun Gopal

*Veterinary Clinics of North America: Food Animal Practice* (ISSN 0749-0720) is published in March, July, and November by Elsevier Inc., 360 Park Avenue South, New York, NY 10010-1710. Subscription prices are $281.00 per year (domestic individuals), $100.00 per year (domestic students/residents), $298.00 per year (Canadian individuals), $356.00 per year (international individuals) $100.00 per year (Canadian students), and $165.00 (international students). For institutional access pricing please contact Customer Service via the contact information below. To receive student/ resident rate, orders must be accompanied by name of affiliated institution, date of term, and the signature of program/ residency coordinator on institution letterhead. *Clinics* subscription prices. All prices are subject to change without notice. **POSTMASTER:** Send address changes to *Veterinary Clinics of North America*: *Food Animal Practice*, Elsevier Health Sciences Division, Subscription Customer Service, 3251 Riverport Lane, Maryland Heights, MO 63043. Customer Service (orders, claims, online, change of address): Elsevier Health Sciences Division, Subscription **Customer Service, 3251 Riverport Lane, Maryland Heights, MO 63043. Tel: 1-800-654-2452 (U.S. and Canada); 314-447-8871 (ouside U.S. and Canada). Fax: 314-447-8029. E-mail: journalscustomerservice-usa@elsevier.com (for print support); journalsonlinesupport-usa@elsevier.com (for online support).**

*Reprints.* For copies of 100 or more, of articles in this publication, please contact the Commercial Reprints Department, Elsevier Inc., 360 Park Avenue South, New York, NY 10010-1710. Tel.: 212-633-3874; Fax: 212-633-3820; E-mail: reprints@elsevier.com.

*Veterinary Clinics of North America: Food Animal Practice* is covered in *Current Contents/Agriculture, Biology and Environmental Sciences, MEDLINE/PubMed (Index Medicus), and Excerpta Medica.*

# Contributors

## CONSULTING EDITOR

**ROBERT A. SMITH, DVM, MS**
Diplomate, American Board of Veterinary Practitioners; Veterinary Research and Consulting Services, LLC, Greeley, Colorado; Veterinary Research and Consulting Services, LLC, Stillwater, Oklahoma

## EDITORS

**ARTHUR LEE JONES, DVM, MS**
Associate Professor, Department of Population Health, UGA College of Veterinary Medicine, UGA TVDIL, Tifton, Georgia; Senior Professional Services Veterinarian - Beef, Boehringer-Ingelheim Animal Health, Duluth, Georgia

**JOSEPH C. DALTON, PhD**
Professor, Extension Dairy Specialist, Animal, Veterinary and Food Sciences Department, University of Idaho, Caldwell, Idaho

## AUTHORS

**CHANCE L. ARMSTRONG, DVM, MS**
Diplomate, American College of Theriogenologists; Associate Clinical Professor of Theriogenology, Auburn University College of Veterinary Medicine, Auburn, Alabama

**AUBREY N. BAIRD, DVM, MS**
Diplomate, American College of Veterinary Surgeons; Associate Dean for Clinical Affairs, Auburn University College of Veterinary Medicine, Auburn, Alabama

**LEONARDO F.C. BRITO, DVM, PhD**
Diplomate, American College of Theriogenologists; Department of Clinical Studies - New Bolton Center, University of Pennsylvania School of Veterinary Medicine, Kennett Square, Pennsylvania

**JOSEPH C. DALTON, PhD**
Professor, Extension Dairy Specialist, Animal, Veterinary and Food Sciences Department, University of Idaho, Caldwell, Idaho

**RICHARD M. HOPPER, DVM**
Diplomate, American College of Theriogenologists; Professor of Theriogenology, Department of Clinical Sciences, College of Veterinary Medicine, Auburn University, Auburn, Alabama

**ARTHUR LEE JONES, DVM, MS**
Associate Professor, Department of Population Health, UGA College of Veterinary Medicine, UGA TVDIL, Tifton, Georgia; Senior Professional Services Veterinarian - Beef, Boehringer-Ingelheim Animal Health, Duluth, Georgia

**E. HEATH KING, DVM, MS**
Diplomate, American College of Theriogenologists; Associate Clinical Professor, Theriogenology, Department of Pathobiology and Population Medicine, College of Veterinary Medicine, Mississippi State University, Mississippi State, Mississippi

**JENNIFER H. KOZIOL, DVM, MS**
Diplomate, American College of Theriogenologists; Associate Professor of Food Animal Medicine and Surgery, Texas Tech School of Veterinary Medicine, Amarillo, Texas

**GRAHAM CLIFF LAMB, MS, PhD**
Professor; Director of Texas A&M Agrilife Research, College Station, Texas

**KELSEY N. LOCKHART, MS**
Division of Animal Sciences, University of Missouri, Columbia, Missouri

**VITOR R.G. MERCADANTE, DVM, MS, PhD**
Affiliate Assistant Professor, School of Animal Sciences, CALS and Large Animal Clinical Sciences, VAMD-CVM at Virginia Tech, Blacksburg, Virginia

**RAMIRO VANDER OLIVEIRA FILHO, PhD**
Department of Animal Science, Pregnancy and Developmental Programming Area of Excellence, Texas A&M University, College Station, Texas

**M. SOFIA ORTEGA, PhD**
Assistant Professor, Department of Animal and Dairy Sciences, University of Wisconsin-Madison, Madison, Wisconsin

**JOE C. PASCHAL, PhD**
Executive Vice President, American Brahman Breeders Association, Bryan, Texas

**FRANCISCO PEÑAGARICANO, PhD**
Assistant Professor, Department of Animal and Dairy Sciences, University of Wisconsin-Madison, Madison, Wisconsin

**GEORGE A. PERRY, PhD**
Professor, Texas A&M AgriLife Research and Extension Center, Overton, Texas

**KY G. POHLER, PhD**
Assistant Professor, Department of Animal Science, Pregnancy and Developmental Programming Area of Excellence, Texas A&M University, College Station, Texas

**THOMAS E. SPENCER, PhD**
Professor, Division of Animal Sciences, University of Missouri, Columbia, Missouri

**GARY D. WARNER, DVM**
Elgin Veterinary Hospital, Elgin, Texas

# Contents

> This manuscript provides an overview of the effects of nutrition during different stages of bull sexual development. Nutrition during the prepubertal period can modulate the hypothalamic GnRH pulse generator. Increased nutrition results in greater LH secretion, earlier puberty, and greater testicular mass in yearling bulls, whereas low nutrition has opposite effects. Targeting average daily gain from birth to 24 weeks of age to > 1.2 kg/d and limiting gain after 24 weeks of age to < 1.6 kg/d is recommended to optimize bull sexual development.

> Physical evaluation of beef bulls is important in determining their ability to be long-lived useful breeding animals. A basic examination should include an assessment of the bull's conformation, gait, and overall appearance. Skeletal soundness can be easily evaluated with well-formed feet and legs. Muscularity and reproductive soundness can be verified visually as should the head and mouth. Finally, attention should be paid to breed characteristics if it is a purebred bull. A bull must be able to walk, eat, and see to effectively function as a natural service sire in pasture, pens, or especially extensive range environments.

> Breeding soundness for several reasons and at several times during their life span. These include before sale for the reason of affirming their sale ability or before a breeding season to determine their readiness for breeding. Bulls may also be evaluated for diagnostic purposes. The breeding soundness examination (BSE) is universally promoted as an important management tool, but there continues to be a level of inconsistency in its performance. A complete bull BSE consists of a thorough physical examination including internal and external reproductive tract, measurement of the circumference of the scrotum and evaluation of individual sperm motility and morphology.

Semen morphology evaluation in the field should always be performed at 1000× with oil immersion. The development of a spermiogram will aid the practitioner to interpret potential fertility of semen at the time of sampling as well as determine potential causes of an abnormal spermiogram. Bulls, which experience stress or impairment of thermoregulation of the testes for any reason, often experience a transitory decrease in the quality of sperm morphology. This can be recognized by a sequence of appearances of morphologic defects coupled with a thorough patient history.

The cause of subfertility or poor fertility in naturally mated bulls should be differentiated from impotentia coeundi, generandi, or erigendi prior to ancillary semen evaluation. Bulls used for artificial insemination may undergo ancillary semen evaluation following low fertility rates as judged by poor conception or low pregnancy rates. Morphologically abnormal sperm have long been associated with bull subfertility and infertility. Some morphological defects such as improper sperm chromatin condensation are not visible using traditional light microscopy and require specialized staining. Ancillary semen evaluation is useful in cases where the reason for low or absence of fertility needs to be identified. As compared to SEM, TEM can be extremely useful for identifying minuscule acrosome defects, issues with chromatin, and centrosome defects and is considered the gold standard method for the identification of midpiece and tail defects.

The inability of a bull to reproduce due to its inability to impregnant fertile cows is called *impotentia generandi*. This infertility may be due to the inability to achieve erection, the inability to complete coitus, or the inability to produce an adequate volume of morphologically normal spermatozoa. Therapies targeting the urogenital tract of the bull can restore reproductive capabilities. Veterinarians can provide consultation regarding both management and selection criteria that will, in some cases, lower the overall risk of loss associated with the development of some conditions of the penis and prepuce.

Abnormalities of the bovine scrotum and testes are an important cause of infertility. Proper evaluation of the male reproductive system is a critical first step in screening for such abnormalities. Excessive periscrotal fat, cutaneous scrotal defects, and unilateral scrotal swelling are common deformities that warrant further investigation. Early diagnosis and surgical intervention are often needed to restore reproductive soundness. This article reviews these conditions and provides therapeutic modalities.

Lameness in bulls is a common problem seen by many veterinarians, and the cause can be difficult to determine. Understanding cattle lameness requires experience and complete knowledge of their structural anatomy and handling. This article reviews the common body regions that cause lameness in bulls and discusses their treatment. It also details hoof trimming as a way to manage lameness.

Reproduction is essential for successful cow-calf and dairy production and the most important economic trait for cow-calf producers. For efficient reproduction to occur in beef herds, cows or heifers must conceive early during the breeding season, maintain the pregnancy, calve unassisted or with very little assistance, rebred in a timely manner and wean a calf every year. In the case of dairy cattle, cows or heifers are expected to become pregnant, maintain the pregnancy, and calve every 12 to 15 months to produce milk. Interruption of that process leads to delay or total loss of production. Although fertile bulls are required to achieve reproduction, they come with potential risk of transmitting disease during breeding.

For over a century, scientists have attempted to develop techniques to accurately predict the fertility potential of a male's semen sample. In most livestock species, the sire is responsible for multiple pregnancies per year and up to hundreds of thousands of pregnancies if used for artificial insemination. Use of subfertile or infertile sires can have devastating impacts in regard to the reproductive efficiency of a cow herd. Despite the rapid expansion of fertility studies through advancements in molecular, genomic, and computer techniques, our understanding of male fertility is still far from complete. This article will provide an overview of the impact of the sire in pregnancy loss.

The use of in vitro embryo production (IVP) has increased globally, particularly in the United States. Although maternal factors influencing embryo development have been extensively studied, the influence of the sire is not well understood. Sperm plays a crucial role in embryo development providing DNA, triggering oocyte maturation, and aiding in mitosis. Current sire fertility measurements do not consistently align with embryo production outcomes. Low-fertility sires may perform well in IVP systems but produce fewer pregnancies. Testing sires in vitro could identify characteristics affecting embryo development and pregnancy loss risk in IVP and embryo transfer programs.

Francisco Peñagaricano

Current evidence suggests that dairy bull fertility is influenced by genetic factors, and hence, it could be managed and improved by genetic means. There are major mutations that explain about 4% to 8% of the observed differences in conception rate between bulls segregating in most dairy breeds. Research has shown that genomic prediction of bull fertility is possible, and this could be used to make accurate genome-guided selection decisions, such as early culling of predicted subfertile bull calves. Inbreeding negatively influences bull fertility, and the increase in homozygosity seems an important risk factor for dairy bull subfertility.

# VETERINARY CLINICS OF NORTH AMERICA: FOOD ANIMAL PRACTICE

# Preface

# Reproduction in Beef and Dairy Herds: From the Male's Perspective

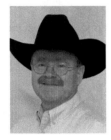
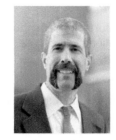

Arthur Lee Jones, DVM, MS      Joseph C. Dalton, PhD
*Editors*

Bulls, whether through natural service (NS) or artificial insemination (AI), contribute to reproductive efficiency and genetic advancement of beef and dairy herds. Today, most dairies and some beef operations rely heavily on the use of AI to breed cows and heifers. How producers and veterinarians manage the male (NS and AI) in each production system impacts reproductive success, as each approach has unique considerations. In addition, we want to provide up-to-date information regarding (a) the contribution of sires to success or failure of reproductive programs in beef and dairy herds, and (b) the foundational material for success with AI (semen storage, handling, and site of deposition).

Veterinarians play an essential role in the initial evaluation of yearling bulls for potential fertility as well as in maintaining the health and function of herd bulls to assure a high percentage of cows and heifers exposed become pregnant and produce a viable calf. A goal of this issue is to provide practitioners with the most current information available to assess the reproductive potential of bulls. In the articles entitled "Physical Evaluation of Beef Bulls," "The Bull Breeding Soundness Examination and its Application in the Production Setting," and "Field Morphology and Interpretation," practitioners are provided with essential criteria to evaluate yearling bulls for future fertility and function. The articles, "Medical and Surgical Management of Conditions of the Penis and Prepuce" and "Bovine Lameness from the Ground Up," provide practitioners with practical resources to diagnose disease or causes of infertility and determine appropriate course of treatment or prognosis for recovery of injured bulls from some of our profession's leading experts. In the article, "Sexually Transmitted Diseases of Bulls," the bull's role in spreading reproductive diseases is explored as well as methods to diagnose and

Vet Clin Food Anim 40 (2024) xi–xii
https://doi.org/10.1016/j.cvfa.2023.10.001
0749-0720/24/© 2023 Published by Elsevier Inc.

mitigate effects of infectious causes of infertility. In the articles entitled, "Implementing Fixed-Time Artificial Insemination Programs in Beef Herds," "Frozen Bovine Semen Storage, Semen Handling, and Site of Deposition," and "Considerations for Using Natural Service with Estrous Synchronization Programs," factors impacting the success of implementing estrus synchronization and AI programs are discussed. Other articles explore effects of sires on fertility and pregnancy success.

Although bull management during the nonbreeding season is critical to successful breeding season performance, few articles exist describing best management practices recommended between breeding seasons. "Managing Beef Bulls During the Off-Season" summarizes some of the current considerations for managing bulls for optimal reproductive performance.

It's our hope this issue will be a useful resource for busy practitioners to assist them in providing up-to-date recommendations and services to their clients.

## CONFLICT OF INTEREST/DISCLOSURES

A. L. Jones does not have any conflicts of interest to disclose. No funds were used in the writing of these articles. J. C. Dalton does not have any conflicts of interest to disclose. No funds were used in the writing of these articles.

Arthur Lee Jones, DVM, MS
Boehringer-Ingelheim Animal Health
3239 Satellite Boulevard NW, Duluth, GA, USA

5012 Georgia Highway 125 North
Chula, GA 31733, USA

Joseph C. Dalton, PhD
Animal, Veterinary and Food Sciences Department
University of Idaho
1904 East Chicago Street, Suite AB
Caldwell, ID 83605, USA

*E-mail addresses:*
lee.jones@boehringer-ingelheim.com (A.L. Jones)
jdalton@uidaho.edu (J.C. Dalton)

# Nutrition and Sexual Development in Bulls

Leonardo F.C. Brito, DVM, PhD

## KEYWORDS

- Bull • Nutrition • Puberty • Testis • Spermatogenesis

## KEY POINTS

- Nutrition during the prepubertal period can modulate the hypothalamic GnRH pulse generator in bulls.
- Increased nutrition during the prepubertal results in greater LH secretion, earlier puberty, and greater testicular mass in yearling bulls, whereas low nutrition has opposite effects.
- The beneficial effects of high nutrition during the prepubertal period extend beyond 24 weeks of age, but the deleterious effects of low nutrition cannot be compensated by high nutrition.
- High-energy diets after the prepubertal period have been associated with low sperm production and poor semen quality.

## INTRODUCTION

Sexual development is of crucial importance for cattle production efficiency. The ability to breed animals at younger ages reduces generation intervals and increases genetic gains. However, delayed puberty, reduced sperm production, and poor semen quality due to immaturity are common causes of poor reproductive performance in young bulls. Therefore, an understanding of the factors that affect sexual development is required to promote the successful use of young bulls for reproductive purposes. The objective of this article is to review the mechanisms by which nutrition affects bull sexual development.

## THE METABOLIC SENSOR

The mechanisms controlling nutrition and reproduction are intrinsically related and have evolved to confer reproductive advantages and to guarantee the survival of the species. The neural apparatus designed to gauge metabolic rate and energy balance by the body has been denominated "metabolic sensor." This sensor translates signals provided by circulating (peripheral) concentrations of specific hormones into

Department of Clinical Studies - New Bolton Center, University of Pennsylvania School of Veterinary Medicine, 382 West Street Road, Kennett Square, PA 19348, USA
*E-mail address:* lbrito@vet.upenn.edu

Vet Clin Food Anim 40 (2024) 1–10
https://doi.org/10.1016/j.cvfa.2023.08.002

neuronal signals that ultimately regulate the gonadotropin-releasing hormone (GnRH) pulse generator and control reproductive function.[1,2]

The bovine somatotropic axis (growth hormone [GH]/insulin-like growth factor-I [IGF-I]) becomes activated in late fetal life or very shortly after birth. Although hepatic growth hormone receptor (GHR) is absent in bovine fetuses up to 8 months of gestation, GHR is expressed in the liver of 1-day-old calves. In addition, IGF-I release in response to GH challenge has been demonstrated in calves within the first week after birth.[3] Growth hormone concentrations decrease during the pubertal period in bulls.[4,5] The GH profile in bulls seems to indicate that a relatively advanced stage of body development must be attained before the gonads are efficiently producing sperm.

IGF-I is primarily synthesized by the liver in response to GH and seems to play a crucial role in the sexual development of bulls. Circulating IGF-I concentrations in bulls increase continuously with age and only reach a plateau (or decrease slightly) after development is mostly completed at 12 to 14 months of age.[4–7] Circulating concentrations of IGF-binding protein 3 (IGFBP-3) increase and concentrations of IGF-binding protein 2 decrease with age, reflecting a likely increase in IGF-I bioavailability.[8,9] Circulating testosterone concentration greater than 2 ng/mL was attained when IGF-I was greater than 150 ng/mL[10] and puberty was attained when IGF-I was greater than 550 ng/mL.[5] Increasing IGF-I concentrations with concomitant decreasing GH concentrations suggest that maximum responsiveness of the GH/IGF-I system and optimization of metabolic regulation and physiologic growth is important for sexual development in bulls.

Increased liver sensitivity to GH due to GHR upregulation is the most likely mechanism by which circulating IGF-I concentrations increase in growing bulls, although production by other organs might also be important. The testes are a possible source of IGF-I because Leydig cells can secrete this hormone in other species. Observations that intact bulls tend to have greater IGF-I concentrations than castrated steers at 12 months of age further support the hypothesis that the testes might contribute substantially to circulating IGF-I concentrations during the prepubertal and pubertal periods in bulls.[11]

Circulating IGF-I and IGF-binding protein (IGFBP-3) concentrations are reduced when cattle experience negative energy balance, like for example, in the postpartum with beginning of lactation or in undernourished animals.[8] Plasma IGF-I concentrations before and after GH challenge differed between bull calves gaining 0.95 to 1.4 kg/d from 1 to 15 weeks of age and calves gaining 0.5 kg/d. Although plasma IGF-I concentrations increased during the first 15 weeks of age, nutrition effects on IGF-I were more pronounced than age.[3] Negative effects of low nutrition and positive effects of high nutrition associated with different circulating IGF-I concentrations have also been demonstrated at different stages of sexual development in bulls up to approximately 1.5 years of age.[4,6,12,13] These observations indicate that IGF-I is a sensitive system to signal metabolic status to the central nervous system (CNS) and peripheral organs.

IGF-I involvement in the regulation of GnRH secretion seems to be an important, conserved physiologic mechanism of metabolic status signaling with accumulating supporting evidence from in vitro and vivo studies in several mammalian species in both males and females.[14–16] Insulin-like growth factor-I receptors (IGF-IR) are highly concentrated within the median eminence of the hypothalamus. IGF-I seems to bind to IGF-IR in glial cells and stimulate the release of prostaglandin-E2, which binds to its receptors on nearby GnRH nerve terminals and causes GnRH release. In female rodents and primates, prepubertal increase in serum IGF-I followed by elevated hypothalamic-pituitary-ovarian activity demonstrates the general influence of IGF-I to facilitate GnRH secretion and the pubertal process.[15,17,18]

Metabolic hormones may also have direct effects on the testes. IGF-IR has been identified in Leydig cells, Sertoli cells, and at least some germ cell types. IGF-I has been shown to affect testicular differentiation, Sertoli cell proliferation, and germ cell proliferation and differentiation in several species. In addition, IGF-I, through PI3K/ AKT signaling, seems to be required for follicle-stimulating hormone (FSH) action.[19–22] In bulls, circulating IGF-I concentrations were associated with scrotal circumference and paired-testes weight in young, growing bulls.[4,5] Sertoli cells from 8-week-old calves show greater in vitro proliferation when exposed to a combination of IGF-I and FSH than when treated with either IGF-I or FSH alone, suggesting an important interaction between IGF-I and FSH in Sertoli cell differentiation and proliferation in bulls.[23]

## SEXUAL DEVELOPMENT

The process of sexual development in bulls involves a complex maturation mechanism of the hypothalamus-pituitary-testes axis. Timing of sexual development is determined primarily by the hypothalamus and GnRH secretion. The infantile period of sexual development is characterized by low gonadotropin and testosterone secretion and relatively few changes in testicular cellular composition. This period extends from birth until approximately 8 weeks of age. The prepubertal period is characterized by a temporary increase in gonadotropin secretion, the so-called early gonadotropin rise, which is associated with dramatic changes in testicular cellular composition, initial increase in testosterone secretion, and timing of attainment of puberty. This period extends from approximately 8 to 24 weeks of age in bulls. The pubertal period of sexual development is characterized by reduced gonadotropin secretion, increased testosterone secretion, initiation of spermatogenesis, and the eventual appearance of sperm in the ejaculate. This period also coincides with the start of a phase of rapid testicular growth and extends from approximately 6 to 12 months of age.[24,25]

The crucial role of the early gonadotropin rise, especially luteinizing hormone (LH) secretion pattern, in regulating sexual development in bulls has been well documented. Luteinizing hormone secretion was greater from 10 to 20 weeks of age in early maturing beef bulls than in late-maturing beef bulls.[26,27] Hormonal treatment to decrease LH secretion from 6 to 14 weeks of age resulted in delayed puberty, reduced testicular weight and number of germ cells in tubular cross-sections at 50 weeks of age.[28] On the other hand, treatment with GnRH every 2 hours from 4 to 6 weeks of age increased LH pulse frequency and mean concentration, testosterone concentration, scrotal circumference, paired-testes weight, seminiferous tubule diameter, and number of germ and Sertoli cells in tubular cross-sections at 54 weeks of age.[29] The accelerated testicular growth observed after 24 weeks of age in bulls occurs when circulating gonadotropins concentrations are decreasing, which points to the existence of important GnRH-independent mechanisms regulating testicular development. Testicular growth involves increases in seminiferous tubule diameter and length, volume of testicular parenchyma occupied by seminiferous tubules, and total number of germ cells.[30]

## NUTRITION DURING THE INFANTILE AND PREPUBERTAL PERIODS (BIRTH TO 24 WEEKS)

The effect of different diets fed only during the infantile period on long-term sexual development in bulls has not been extensively studied but recent data suggest that poor nutrition might result in detrimental decoupling of the somatotropic axis early in life, whereas increased nutrition during the infantile period might have long-term, beneficial effects on subsequent reproductive performance of bull calves.

Holstein bull calves fed to gain 1.28 kg/d during the first 3 weeks of age had relatively low circulating GH but elevated IGF-I concentrations, indicating maximal responsiveness of the somatotropic system and optimal physiologic growth. In contrast, calves fed to gain 0.38 kg/d had marginal IGF-I concentration irrespective of high GH concentrations. Although calves received the same diet after 4 weeks of age, circulating testosterone concentrations were greater in bulls that had received high nutrition.[31] In Brown Swiss bull calves, greater milk intake during the first 4 weeks of age was associated with greater circulating testosterone concentrations between 24 and 52 weeks of age and with greater production of morphologically normal sperm between 40 and 64 weeks of age.[32]

Differences in yearling scrotal circumference due to age of the dam in beef bulls could be interpreted as an indication that nutrition during the infantile and prepubertal periods affects sexual development. Scrotal circumference in beef bulls increases as age of the dam increases until 5 to 9 years of age and decreases as dams get older.[33,34] The effect of age of the dam on testicular growth seems to be primarily the result of the bull's body weight, likely related to differences in milk intake. This theory is also supported by reports that, similarly to that observed in bulls receiving low nutrition, LH secretion after GnRH challenge was lower from 14 to 24 weeks of age in beef bulls raised by first-lactation cows than in bulls raised by multiparous cows.[35]

Low nutrition during the prepubertal period reduces LH pulse secretion by delaying the early gonadotropin increase, decreasing the number of daily LH pulses, or both. However, high nutrition during this stage of development hastens the early gonadotrophin increase, sustains increased LH pulsatile secretion for a longer period of time, or both. The LH secretion pattern during the prepubertal period is associated with sexual development including testicular growth, testosterone secretion, and sperm production. Lower LH secretion in bulls receiving low nutrition during the prepubertal period is associated with delayed testosterone secretion, increased age at puberty, and smaller yearling testes weight. Bulls receiving high nutrition have greater LH secretion, reach puberty earlier, and have greater testicular mass. Results from GnRH challenges revealed that differences in LH pulse secretion in bulls receiving different nutrition are not necessarily associated with reduced pituitary LH secretion capacity.[4,6,36] Therefore, nutrition seems to have a direct effect on the GnRH pulse generator in the hypothalamus. However, LH secretion after GnRH challenge might also be diminished in bulls fed low nutrition, indicating that in some cases nutrition effects might also extend beyond the hypothalamus.[7,12] No nutrition effect on circulating FSH has been reported in bulls.[4,6,13]

Close temporal associations observed in several studies suggest that circulating IGF-I concentrations modulates the GnRH pulse generator and the magnitude and duration of the early gonadotropin rise in bulls. Circulating GH, insulin, and leptin concentrations, however, did not differ among bull calves receiving different prepubertal nutrition; therefore, the role of these hormones in regulating GnRH secretion, if any, seems to be at most permissive. Nutrition also affected testicular steroidogenesis (ie, testosterone concentrations), reflecting effects on number of Leydig cells, cell function, or both. The increase in physiologic and GnRH-stimulated circulating testosterone concentrations observed with age was hastened in bulls receiving high nutrition and delayed in bulls receiving low nutrition. Because LH and IGF-I have crucial complementary roles in promoting Leydig cell proliferation, differentiation, and testosterone secretion, it can be speculated that the effects of nutrition on testicular steroidogenesis were probably mediated by both LH secretion and IGF-I concentrations.[4,6,12,13,36–38]

Genome-wide analysis of testicular tissue has provided further support that nutrition during the prepubertal period significantly affects sexual development. Testicular gene expression did not differ between Holstein bulls receiving low or high nutrition during the infantile period (before 8 weeks of age) or after the prepubertal period (32 weeks of age).[39] However, several genes were upregulated in the high nutrition group at 16 and 24 weeks of age. Genes with the greatest difference between groups included FDX1, HMGCR, HMGCS1, ACSS2, and PRUNE2 at 16 weeks and KRT8, ENPP3, CA3, and HSD17B3 at 24 weeks of age. Enriched pathways in the high nutrition group included "cholesterol biosynthesis," "steroid metabolism," and "glutamine and creatinine biosynthesis." Functional analysis revealed enhanced lipid, vitamin, and mineral metabolism. Downregulated genes at 24 weeks in the high-nutrition group included AMH and DPT, both negative regulators of cell proliferation.[39]

Bulls fed high nutrition until 24 weeks of age had greater sperm production and sperm motility between 32 and 60 weeks of age than bulls fed with low nutrition.[37] Testicular gene expression at 72 weeks of age did not differ between bulls receiving low or medium nutrition starting at 2 weeks of age. However, hundreds of genes involved in oxidative phosphorylation and mitochondrial protein synthesis were upregulated in bulls receiving high nutrition.[40] Nutrition during the prepubertal period might also have long-term effects on sperm epigenetics. When sperm were obtained after 55 weeks of age from bulls fed low nutrition from 2 to 32 weeks of age, hypermethylation of several regions of the genome was observed. Major genes included some in the mitogen-activated protein kinase signaling pathway (AKT1, AKT2, EGFR, and MAPK1) and some associated with spermatogenesis and sperm function (CYP26B1, DDX4, SPATA13, EQTN, and DNMT3a). Dynamic changes in the sperm epigenome associated with prepubertal nutrition could potentially affect sperm function, embryonic development, and fertility.[41]

The effects of nutrition during the prepubertal period, either the deleterious effects of low nutrition or the beneficial effects of high nutrition, are largely independent from the nutrition during the pubertal period. Studies have shown that, regardless of the nutrition offered after 24 weeks of age, bulls receiving low nutrition from approximately 8 to 24 weeks of age are approximately 3 to 4 weeks older at puberty. However, paired-testis weight is 50 to 120 g greater at 1.5 years of age in bulls receiving high nutrition.[12,13,36,37] These studies demonstrate that the prepubertal period is the most important when considering different nutritional strategies for prospective breeding bulls.

## NUTRITION AFTER THE PREPUBERTAL PERIOD

Similarly to that observed in the prepubertal period, there is considerable evidence to suggest that low nutrition after the prepubertal period has negative effects on reproductive function. In a series of experiments, beef bulls aged 32 to 48 weeks receiving diets with low levels of crude protein (1.5%–8%) for periods of 3 to 6 months had markedly reduced testes, epididymides, and seminal gland weights when compared with control bulls fed with diets containing 14% crude protein. Moreover, seminiferous tubule diameter and seminiferous epithelium thickness were smaller in bulls with restricted protein intake.[42,43] Likewise, 20-month-old Bos indicus and crossbred bulls fed to gain only 0.3 kg/d for 12 months had significantly lower scrotal circumference, testes and epididymides weight, daily sperm production, and epididymal sperm reserves than bulls fed to gain 0.8 kg/d.[44]

Contrary to low nutrition, high nutrition after the prepubertal period does not seem to promote sexual maturation or improve sperm production. In a study with beef bulls evaluated between 24 weeks and 1.5 years of age, no significant correlations were observed between average daily gain (1–1.6 kg/d) and age at puberty, scrotal circumference, testes weight, daily sperm production, or epididymal sperm reserves.[45] Bulls receiving high nutrition in the pubertal period after receiving low nutrition in the prepubertal period had quick compensatory weight gain but were still older at puberty and had smaller testes than bulls fed adequately during the peripubertal period.[12,37] These results indicate that high nutrition during the pubertal period cannot "compensate" for previous nutritional deficiencies.

In fact, diets that promote excessive weight gain during the pubertal period adversely affect sperm production and semen quality. High-energy postweaning diets are frequently associated with impaired reproductive function due to impaired testicular thermoregulation. Sperm motility decreased and the proportion of sperm defects increased with age in beef bulls fed to gain greater than 1.75 kg/d after 76 weeks of age when compared with bulls fed to gain 1 kg/d. There was greater deposition of fat around the testicular vascular cone in the scrotal neck in bulls in the high-nutrition group, which likely resulted in increased testicular temperature.[46]

In a series of experiments with beef bulls fed high nutrition (80% grain and 20% forage) or medium nutrition (forage only) from 24 weeks to 1 to 2 years of age, bulls receiving high nutrition had greater body weight and back fat but testes weight was not affected by diet. Moreover, bulls receiving high nutrition had lower daily sperm production and epididymal sperm reserves, and greater proportion of sperm abnormalities. Increased dietary energy was also associated with increased scrotal skin temperature.[47–50] Another interesting observation is that bulls fed high-nutrition diets had greater scrotal circumference (SC) than bulls fed medium-nutrition diets but testes weight was the same. However, scrotal weight was greater in bulls fed with high nutrition, suggesting that fat deposition in the scrotum was likely responsible for the greater SC obtained in these bulls.[51]

The accelerated testicular growth after the prepubertal period coincides with increasing circulating IGF-I and leptin concentrations and strong associations between these hormones and testicular size have been observed in growing beef bulls, indicating that metabolic hormones may be involved in regulating GnRH-independent testicular development.[4,5] Although IGF-I and leptin concentrations were associated with testicular size, there were no associations between these hormones and seminiferous tubule diameter and area, seminiferous epithelium area, or volume occupied by seminiferous tubule (L. Brito, personal observations). These observations suggest that increased circulating IGF-I and leptin concentrations were associated with increased length of the seminiferous tubules and likely with overall increases in the total number of testicular cells. Despite a few publications suggesting a link between insulin and testis development and function, there is no direct evidence to confirm that insulin plays a role in this process.[52]

## SUMMARY

Nutrition's effects on sexual development involve modulation of the hypothalamus-pituitary-testes axis in young bulls. The most profound effect is modulation of the GnRH pulse generator in the hypothalamus until 24 weeks of age. Herein lies the challenge of ensuring that young calves grow to their full genetic potential and also the opportunity to apply targeted, intensive management practices during the first 24 weeks of age to naturally enhance bull reproductive function.

## DISCLOSURE

The author has no affiliations with or involvement in any organization or entity with any financial interest or nonfinancial interest in the subject matter or materials discussed in this article.

## CLINICS CARE POINTS

- Bulls receiving poor nutrition before 24 weeks of age are more likely to experience delayed puberty and to receive unsatisfactory breeding soundness classification as yearlings.
- Over-conditioned bulls receiving high-energy diets are more likely to experience impaired testicular thermoregulation and to produce semen of poor quality with low sperm motility and high percentage of morphologically abnormal sperm.
- Simple recommendations for bull management include targeting average daily gain from birth to 24 weeks of age to >1.2 kg/d and limiting gain after 24 weeks of age to <1.6 kg/d.

## REFERENCES

1. Schneider JE. Energy balance and reproduction. Physiol Behav 2004;81(2): 289–317.
2. Blache D, Zhang S, Martin GB. Fertility in male sheep: modulators of the acute effects of nutrition on the reproductive axis of male sheep. Reprod Suppl 2003; 61:387–402.
3. Smith JM, Van Amburgh ME, Díaz MC, et al. Effect of nutrient intake on the development of the somatotropic axis and its responsiveness to GH in Holstein bull calves1. J Anim Sci 2002;80(6):1528–37.
4. Brito LF, Barth AD, Rawlings NC, et al. Effect of nutrition during calfhood and peripubertal period on serum metabolic hormones, gonadotropins and testosterone concentrations, and on sexual development in bulls. Domest Anim Endocrinol 2007;33(1):1–18.
5. Brito L, Barth A, Rawlings N, et al. Circulating metabolic hormones during the peripubertal period and their association with testicular development in bulls. Reprod Domest Anim 2007;42(5):502–8.
6. Dance A, Thundathil J, Wilde R, et al. Enhanced early-life nutrition promotes hormone production and reproductive development in Holstein bulls. J Dairy Sci 2015;98(2):987–98.
7. Byrne CJ, Fair S, English AM, et al. Effect of breed, plane of nutrition and age on growth, scrotal development, metabolite concentrations and on systemic gonadotropin and testosterone concentrations following a GnRH challenge in young dairy bulls. Theriogenology 2017;96:58–68.
8. Renaville R, Hammadi M, Portetelle D. Role of the somatotropic axis in the mammalian metabolism. Domest Anim Endocrinol 2002;23(1–2):351–60.
9. Renaville R, Van Eenaeme C, Breier BH, et al. Feed restriction in young bulls alters the onset of puberty in relationship with plasma insulin-like growth factor-I (IGF-I) and IGF-binding proteins. Domest Anim Endocrinol 2000;18(2):165–76.
10. Renaville R, Devolder A, Massart S, et al. Changes in the hypophysial-gonadal axis during the onset of puberty in young bulls. J Reprod Fertil 1993;99(2):443–9.
11. Lee CY, Hunt DW, Gray SL, et al. Secretory patterns of growth hormone and insulin-like growth factor-I during peripubertal period in intact and castrate male cattle. Domest Anim Endocrinol 1991;8(4):481–9.
12. Brito LF, Barth AD, Rawlings NC, et al. Effect of feed restriction during calfhood on serum concentrations of metabolic hormones, gonadotropins, testosterone, and on sexual development in bulls. Reproduction 2007;134(1):171–81.
13. Byrne CJ, Fair S, English AM, et al. Plane of nutrition before and after 6 months of age in Holstein-Friesian bulls: II. Effects on metabolic and reproductive

endocrinology and identification of physiological markers of puberty and sexual maturation. J Dairy Sci 2018;101(4):3460–75.

14. Miller BH, Gore AC. Alterations in hypothalamic insulin-like growth factor-I and its associations with gonadotropin releasing hormone neurones during reproductive development and ageing. J Neuroendocrinol 2001;13(8):728–36.

15. Dees WL, Hiney JK, Srivastava VK. IGF-1 Influences Gonadotropin-Releasing Hormone Regulation of Puberty. Neuroendocrinology 2021;111(12):1151–63.

16. Daftary SS, Gore AC. The hypothalamic insulin-like growth factor-1 receptor and its relationship to gonadotropin-releasing hormones neurones during postnatal development. J Neuroendocrinol 2004;16(2):160–9.

17. Olson BR, Scott DC, Wetsel WC, et al. Effects of insulin-like growth factors I and II and insulin on the immortalized hypothalamic GTI-7 cell line. Neuroendocrinology 1995;62(2):155–65.

18. Anderson RA, Zwain IH, Arroyo A, et al. The insulin-like growth factor system in the GT1-7 GnRH neuronal cell line. Neuroendocrinology 1999;70(5):353–9.

19. Wang G, Hardy MP. Development of leydig cells in the insulin-like growth factor-I (igf-I) knockout mouse: effects of igf-I replacement and gonadotropic stimulation. Biol Reprod 2004;70(3):632–9.

20. Villalpando I, Lira E, Medina G, et al. Insulin-like growth factor 1 is expressed in mouse developing testis and regulates somatic cell proliferation. Experimental biology and medicine 2008;233(4):419–26.

21. Escott GM, de Castro AL, Jacobus AP, et al. Insulin and IGF-I actions on IGF-I receptor in seminiferous tubules from immature rats. Biochimica et Biophysica Acta (BBA)-Biomembranes 2014;1838(5):1332–7.

22. Cannarella R, Condorelli R, La Vignera S, et al. Effects of the insulin-like growth factor system on testicular differentiation and function: a review of the literature. Andrology 2018;6(1):3–9.

23. Dance A, Kastelic J, Thundathil J. A combination of insulin-like growth factor I (IGF-I) and FSH promotes proliferation of prepubertal bovine Sertoli cells isolated and cultured in vitro. Reprod Fertil Dev 2017;29(8):1635–41.

24. Amann RP. Endocrine changes associated with onset of spermatogenesis in Holstein bulls. J Dairy Sci 1983;66(12):2606–22.

25. Rawlings NC, Fletcher PW, Henricks DM, et al. Plasma luteinizing hormone (LH) and testosterone levels during sexual maturation in beef bull calves. Biol Reprod 1978;19(5):1108–12.

26. Aravindakshan JP, Honaramooz A, Bartlewski PM, et al. Pattern of gonadotropin secretion and ultrasonographic evaluation of developmental changes in the testis of early and late maturing bull calves. Theriogenology 2000;54(3):339–54.

27. Evans A, Davies F, Nasser L, et al. Differences in early patterns of gonadotrophin secretion between early and late maturing bulls, and changes in semen characteristics at puberty. Theriogenology 1995;43:569–78.

28. Chandolia RK, Evans AC, Rawlings NC. Effect of inhibition of increased gonadotrophin secretion before 20 weeks of age in bull calves on testicular development. J Reprod Fertil 1997;109(1):65–71.

29. Chandolia RK, Honaramooz A, Bartlewski PM, et al. Effects of treatment with LH releasing hormone before the early increase in LH secretion on endocrine and reproductive development in bull calves. J Reprod Fertil 1997;111(1):41–50.

30. Curtis SK, Amann RP. Testicular development and establishment of spermatogenesis in Holstein bulls. J Anim Sci 1981;53(6):1645–57.

31. Maccari P, Wiedemann S, Kunz HJ, et al. Effects of two different rearing protocols for Holstein bull calves in the first 3 weeks of life on health status, metabolism and subsequent performance. J Anim Physiol Anim Nutr 2015;99(4):737–46.
32. Bollwein H, Janett F, Kaske M. Impact of nutritional programming on the growth, health, and sexual development of bull calves. Domest Anim Endocrinol 2016; 56(Suppl):S180–90.
33. Lunstra DD, Gregory KE, Cundiff LV. Heritability estimates and adjustment factors for the effects of bull age and age of dam on yearling testicular size in breeds of bulls. Theriogenology 1988;30(1):127–36.
34. Kriese LA, Bertrand JK, Benyshek LL. Age adjustment factors, heritabilities and genetic correlations for scrotal circumference and related growth traits in Hereford and Brangus bulls. J Anim Sci 1991;69(2):478–89.
35. Bagu E, Davies K, Epp T, et al. The effect of parity of the dam on sexual maturation, serum concentrations of metabolic hormones and the response to luteinizing hormone releasing hormone in bull calves. Reprod Domest Anim 2010;45(5):803–10.
36. Brito LF, Barth AD, Rawlings NC, et al. Effect of improved nutrition during calfhood on serum metabolic hormones, gonadotropins, and testosterone concentrations, and on testicular development in bulls. Domest Anim Endocrinol 2007; 33(4):460–9.
37. Byrne CJ, Fair S, English AM, et al. Plane of nutrition before and after 6 months of age in Holstein-Friesian bulls: I. Effects on performance, body composition, age at puberty, and postpubertal semen production. J Dairy Sci 2018;101(4):3447–59.
38. English AM, Kenny DA, Byrne CJ, et al. Role of early life nutrition on regulating the hypothalamic–anterior pituitary–testicular axis of the bull. Reproduction 2018; 156(4):283–97.
39. Johnson C, Dance A, Kovalchuk I, et al. Enhanced early-life nutrition upregulates cholesterol biosynthetic gene expression and Sertoli cell maturation in testes of pre-pubertal Holstein bulls. Sci Rep 2019;9(1):6448.
40. Johnson C, Dance A, Kovalchuk I, et al. Enhanced pre-pubertal nutrition upregulates mitochondrial function in testes and sperm of post-pubertal Holstein bulls. Sci Rep 2020;10(1):2235.
41. Johnson C, Kiefer H, Chaulot-Talmon A, et al. Prepubertal nutritional modulation in the bull and its impact on sperm DNA methylation. Cell Tissue Res 2022; 389(3):587–601.
42. Meacham T, Warnick A, Cunha T, et al. Hematological and histological changes in young beef bulls fed low protein rations. J Anim Sci 1964;23(2):380–4.
43. Meacham T, Cunha T, Warnick A, et al. Influence of low protein rations on growth and semen characteristics of young beef bulls. J Anim Sci 1963;22(1):115–20.
44. Tegegne A, Dembarga Y, Kassa T. Gonadal and extragonadal sperm reserves in Boran and Boran x Friesian bulls raised on two planes of nutrition in the Highlands of Ethiopia. Theriogenology 1992;37(4):953–61.
45. Brito LF, Barth AD, Wilde RE, et al. Effect of growth rate from 6 to 16 months of age on sexual development and reproductive function in beef bulls. Theriogenology 2012;77(7):1398–405.
46. Skinner J. Nutrition and fertility in pedigree bulls. Environmental factors in mammal reproduction 1981;160–8.
47. Coulter G, Bailey D. Epididymal sperm reserves in 12-month-old Angus and Hereford bulls: Effects of bull strain plus dietary energy. Anim Reprod Sci 1988; 16(3–4):169–75.
48. Coulter G, Carruthers T, Amann R, et al. Testicular development, daily sperm production and epididymal sperm reserves in 15-mo-old Angus and Hereford bulls:

effects of bull strain plus dietary energy. Journal of animal science 1987;64(1): 254–60.

49. Coulter G, Cook R, Kastelic J. Effects of dietary energy on scrotal surface temperature, seminal quality, and sperm production in young beef bulls. J Anim Sci 1997;75(4):1048–52.

50. Coulter G, Kozub G. Testicular development, epididymal sperm reserves and seminal quality in two-year-old Hereford and Angus bulls: effects of two levels of dietary energy. J Anim Sci 1984;59(2):432–40.

51. Seidel Jr G, Pickett B, Wilsey C, et al., Effect of high level of nutrition on reproductive characteristics of Angus bulls. Proceeding of the 9th International Congress on Animal Reproduction and Artificial Insemination 1980.

52. Griffeth RJ, Bianda V, Nef S. The emerging role of insulin-like growth factors in testis development and function. Basic Clin Androl 2014;24:12.

# Physical Evaluation of Beef Bulls

Joe C. Paschal, PhD[a], A. Lee Jones, DVM, MS[b],*

## KEYWORDS

- Bull conformation • Soundness • Physical evaluation

## KEY POINTS

- Bulls must be physically sound to be a successful breeder.
- Some environments require extensive walking, so bulls must be physically able to travel long distances and find cows in estrus.
- A physical evaluation is an essential part of the Bull Breeding Soundness Evaluation.

## INTRODUCTION

Physical evaluation of beef bulls should begin with the size, shape, and position of the feet and legs and observation of the bull at a walk on a firm level surface.[1] Many times, just observing a bull walking on a firm level surface will quickly indicate any issues involving structure. Observation of how a bull places his feet, with the hind feet being placed nearly in or on the prints of the forefeet, is a good indication of structural correctness. Structural correctness is genetically controlled[2] and can be greatly affected by the environment (nutrition and management). It can be altered by corrective actions like hoof trimming, but the cause is still genetic, and extreme structural issues need to be avoided if possible.

## FEET AND LEGS

Begin the evaluation at the base of the bull. The structure of the hooves, feet, and legs is low to moderately heritable,[3,4] and some breeds have scoring systems. However, a simple evaluation often suffices to evaluate correctness. In dairy cattle, there is a positive association between claw conformation, lameness, and longevity.[3]

The toes of the hooves on each foot and on all 4 feet should have the same shape and size. Do not select bulls that have hooves with one toe smaller than the other. Likewise, the shape of the toes on each foot should be similar and the ends of the toes should not cross or lay over the opposite toe on the foot.[4] There should be a

a American Brahman Breeders Association, 1920 West Villa Maria Road #302, Bryan, TX 77807, USA; b Beef Cattle, Boehringer-Ingelheim Animal Health
* Corresponding author. 3239 Satellite Boulevard Northwest, Duluth, GA 30096.
E-mail address: lee.jones@boehringer-ingelheim.com

Vet Clin Food Anim 40 (2024) 11–18
https://doi.org/10.1016/j.cvfa.2023.09.001
0749-0720/24/© 2023 Elsevier Inc. All rights reserved.

moderate amount of interdigital space between the toes to allow the toes of the hoof to spread out while walking and the space between the toes (or digits) need to be free of any corns. However, this interdigital space should not be so wide as to allow the toes to spread out more than about an inch or two.[4] Often toes can be trimmed or shaped (and often are for the show ring) but the genetics for poor foot structure remain.

The toes and hooves of the front feet may be turned out slightly (10–20°) but no wider or the bull will be "splay footed." Likewise, the toes should not be turned inward or they will be "pigeon toed." If a bull is pigeon toed, he is likely to be "knocked kneed," meaning his knees bend inward when seen from in front. If he is splay footed, he is also likely to be "bow legged." The hooves of the hind feet should be parallel to each other, neither turned out nor in (**Fig. 1**).

The heel of the hoof or toe should not rest directly on the ground (**Fig. 2**). The heels of the front and rear feet should be upright to prevent injury to the soft part of the heel. Bulls that walk on their hind feet heels or have weak pasterns are said to be "coon footed" in that they leave a hoof track like a raccoon.

From the side, the rear toes should angle toward the pastern joint at about 45°.[2] Too low of an angle will have the bull walking on the soft part of their heel and too high or steep of an angle will place the bull on their toes and wear them down faster.

From the front of an animal, an imaginary line drawn from the interdigital space between the toes should run through the middle of the lower foreleg, through the middle of the knee, and through the middle of the upper foreleg to a point between the point of the shoulder and middle of the chest. Similarly, with the exception of the slope of the hoof, the foreleg should be straight from the back of the heel to the back of the knee to just in front of the elbow.

Bulls with knee joints that are forward of (buck kneed) or behind (calf kneed) this line have structural issues (**Fig. 3**). Similarly, viewed from the front, the knee joint should

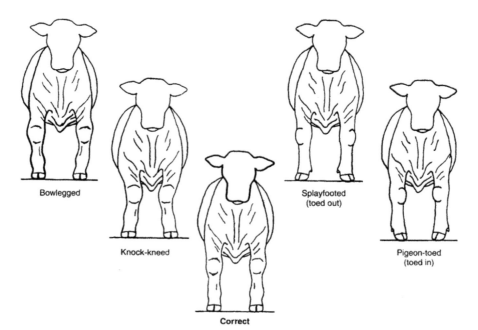

Bowlegged

Knock-kneed

Correct

Splayfooted
(toed out)

Pigeon-toed
(toed in)

**Fig. 1.** Ideal front leg alignment. (*Reproduced from* 4-H Livestock Judging Manual, Mississippi State University Extension publication P2289. [used with permission].)

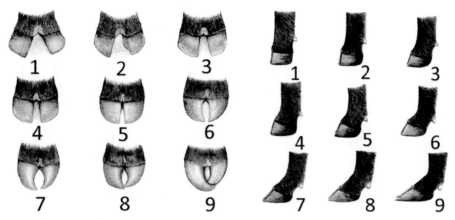

**Fig. 2.** Claw set (left) and Foot angle (right): 5 is ideal. (From Foot Score Guidelines. With permission from American Angus Association. Retrieved from: www.angus.org/performance/Documents/footscorebrochure.pdf.)

not deviate from the center of the leg. When viewed from the side, an imaginary line can be drawn from the base of the heel through the center of the knee up to the elbow joint. At the elbow, the line moves forward to the point of the shoulder and then again at 90° to the base of the shoulder blade. Viewed from above, the tops of the shoulder blades should not be visible (open shouldered) but embedded in muscle.

From the side, front, and rear views, the lower legs should be relatively straight from the pastern to the knee (forelegs) or hock (hind legs). The bull's hocks may be turned in slightly (cow-hocked; **Fig. 4**) but as long as it is not extreme, it is not a defect. Cattle judges prefer a straight hock but it is not natural. Hocks should not be turned out as this presents a "bowlegged" appearance and causes the hind feet to be turned in and may cause more wear on the outer toes. In addition, it is a sign of structural problems.

Viewed from the rear, with the exception of a slight cow hock, a line from the middle of the heel should pass through the middle of the hock to a point halfway between the tail and the outside of the hip (between the pin bone and the hip bone). Bulls with joints that deviate too far from this line have structural problems.

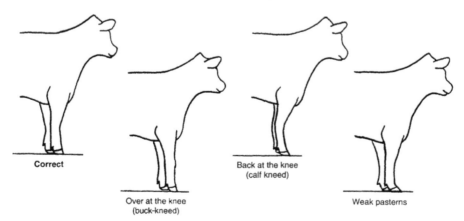

**Fig. 3.** Ideal front leg set. (*Reproduced from* 4-H Livestock Judging Manual, Mississippi State University Extension publication P2289. [used with permission].)

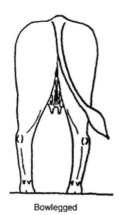
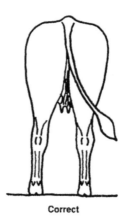
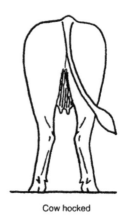

Bowlegged                    Correct                    Cow hocked

**Fig. 4.** Ideal rear leg alignment. (*Reproduced from* 4-H Livestock Judging Manual, Mississippi State University Extension publication P2289. [used with permission].)

From the side (**Fig. 5**), the hind leg will be relatively straight from the back of the heel to the middle of the hock. Too straight of a lower hind limb reduces the cushioning effect of the pastern. From the hock, there should be about a 45° angle to the next joint, the stifle. If this angle is smaller, the bull's hind legs will be tucked under him (sickle hocked) while if this angle is larger, the bull will be too straight legged (post leg). Neither of these conditions is desirable and has the potential to predispose bulls for future lameness.[5,6] Continuing the imaginary line from the stifle to the hip joint is another 45° angle. If any of these are smaller, typically bulls will stand and walk with their feet under their body (sickle hocked) while if any of these angles are larger, the bull will stand with his feet too straight or even behind him. In either case, the pressure on the joints of the hind legs will reduce his breeding soundness over time and sooner than in a bull with more ideal structure.

The width between the hooks should be wide, wider hooks are more desirable than narrow ones since they are an indicator of skeletal frame for muscle mass. The slope and shape of the hip (the line from the hook or hip bones to the pin or tail bones) has always been a point of discussion. Market steer (and some breeding cattle) judges

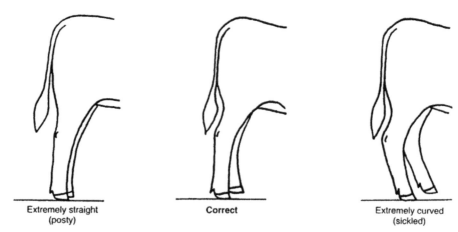

Extremely straight              Correct              Extremely curved
(posty)                                               (sickled)

**Fig. 5.** Ideal feet and leg placement. (*Reproduced from* 4-H Livestock Judging Manual, Mississippi State University Extension publication P2289. [used with permission].)

prefer the shape of the hip to be nearly flat to make a square shape in the show ring but it creates post leggedness which is not ideal in breeding cattle. Breeding cattle need to have a slope of at least 20 (or more) degrees from the hooks to pins to remain structurally correct. Some breeds such as the *Bos indicus* will have a greater slope which some research indicates enhances calving ease.

## SCROTUM

With the feet and leg structure evaluation concluded, there are other areas that need to be considered in physical evaluation even though they may be part of a breeding soundness examination (BSE) or better evaluated by genetic prediction, nevertheless the appearances need to be covered.

Obviously, the reproductive soundness of a bull can be best evaluated by the BSE but if one is not being conducted at the time, bulls should still have a physically acceptable scrotum and sheath. Visible or palpable physical abnormalities of the scrotum decrease the odds of having satisfactory semen qualities.[7–9] The scrotum should contain 2 testicles that are about the same size and shape, neither too hard or too soft, and they should be easily raised and lowered.[7] At the base of the scrotum an enlarged portion should be observed, the epididymis, a storage area for new sperm cells. Sometimes a scrotum can be turned slightly or be different colors (pink or red and black). As long as those bulls pass a BSE, those conditions are cosmetic. Bulls that have *B indicus* genetics tend to have longer scrotums[10,11] to allow the testicles to be lowered further away from the body for cooling while bulls with *B taurus* influence may have shorter scrotums. Excessive pendulousness can predispose bulls to testicle bruising in extensive environments.[9]

## SHEATH

The sheath or skin enclosing the penis should also be evaluated (**Fig. 6**). Most *B taurus* bulls have a relatively tight (close to the body) sheath while *B indicus* bulls (and composite breeds with *B indicus* in them—beefmaster, brangus, santa gertrudis, and other such breeds) will tend to have a looser sheath. Bulls with longer sheaths may also have larger preputial openings allowing the penis and foreskin to "fall out."[9] This can lead to contamination, injury, infection, and failure to breed. Both the size of the sheath and the preputial opening should be considered. It is recommended that the sheath not extend below an imaginary line that extends from the hocks to the knees. Sheath depth has been negatively correlated to calf output.[11] Sheath conformation and umbilical size was also associated with lower serving capacity scores in *B indicus–*influenced bulls in Australia.[11] In another report from Australia, sheath depth in brahman bulls was negatively related to calf output.[9] One final point about the sheath and penis is that the angle of the sheath be less than 45°.

## MUSCLING

There are more precise measures of muscularity than a physical evaluation but it is important to realize where and what to look for muscling. Often only the topline of bulls is evaluated for muscling. This can be deceiving if the bull is too fat and the back will be wide and flat. A bull with good muscling in this area (rib eye and loin) will be rounded and firm and the muscles can be seen to move when the animal walks.

Viewed from the rear, the widest point of the hindquarter should be through the middle of the hind leg and the muscling of the leg should extend downward toward the hock. Well-muscled bulls will stand wide apart as the muscling between their legs

## Sheath characteristics in Brahman and Brahman crossbred bulls

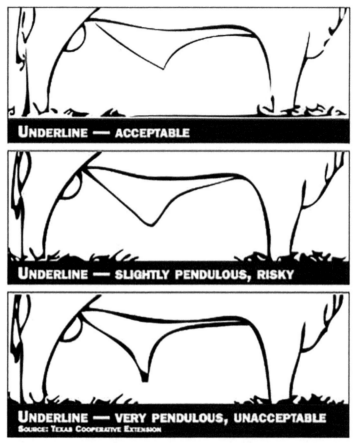

**Fig. 6.** Acceptable sheath characteristics. (From L.R. Sprott, B.B. Carpenter and T.A. Thrift, Bull management for cow/calf producers. B-6064 9/05. With permission from Texas Cooperative Extension archives.)

causes their stance to be widened. From the side, muscling in the hind leg should be evident from the hip or hook bone to the pin bone, across the stifle to above the hock. The muscle in the hind leg will bulge and move when the bull walks.

Similarly, muscling can be easily observed in the front leg below the elbow. The circumference of the forearm is a good indicator of muscling throughout. The circumference of bone in the upper forearm (fused radius and ulna) and the thickness of the skin and subcutaneous fat does not change much in bulls of the same age or breed, so differences in circumference in the upper foreleg indicate differences in muscling throughout. From the front of the bull, a wide chest is also good indicator of muscling.

## HEAD

Although it seems obvious, the head of a bull is often not evaluated extensively. All bulls should have one. A bull should have a wide flat head (due to the influence of testosterone)[12] with two similarly shaped ears. In some *B indicus* bulls, there are reports of a small rudimentary ear on one or both ears that does not affect the performance of the bull but could be a concern to a purebred breeder. The eyes should be clear and of the same size. The pigmentation around the eye in white-faced cattle is preferable to reduce risk of bovine ocular squamous cell carcinoma, cancer eye. The mouth of the bull should have matched upper (no undershot, bulldog, or monkey mouth) and lower (overshot or parrot mouth) jaws; that is, the lower incisors should close on the upper dental pad. The nostrils should be large and similar in size. Bulls can be horned or polled but need to reflect the characteristics of the breed, if purebred.

## HAIR COAT

The hair coat should be free of dead hair or diseased areas and should be uniformly hairy or sleek. Research has shown cattle that shed their winter coat in late spring or early winter have more heat tolerance than cattle that shed later.[12,13] Typically bulls with higher levels of testosterone will be darker in color over their neck and shoulders and sometimes their hindquarters.

## TAIL

Tails are important to prevent insect bites and egg laying. Tails should have a well-formed switch of the color required by the breed, if purebred.

## CREST OR HUMP

Bulls with high levels of testosterone will have a noticeable crest[12] over their neck formed by the enlargement of the trapezius muscle. In *B indicus* cattle and *B indicus*–influenced cattle breeds, this will be greatly enlarged as it is a breed characteristic.

## DISCLOSURE

The authors do not have any conflicts of interests to disclose.

## REFERENCES

1. Alexander J. Evaluation of breeding soundness: the physical examination. In: Hopper RM, editor. Bovine reproduction. 1st edition. Ames, IA: John Wiley and Sons, Inc.; 2015. p. 64–7.
2. Sitz T, Delcurto-Wyffels H, Van Emon M, et al. Importance of foot and leg structure for beef cattle in forage-based production systems. Animals (Basel) 2023;13(3):495.
3. Vermunt J, Greenough P. Hock angles of dairy heifers in two management systems. Br Vet J 1996;152:237–42.
4. McDaniel BT, Verbeek B, Wilk JC, et al. Relationships between hoof measures, stayabilities, reproduction and changes in milk yield from first to later lactations. J Dairy Sci 1984;67:198–9.
5. Figures: 4H Livestock Judging Manual, Mississippi State University Extension. P-2289 4-H Livestock Judging Manual | Mississippi State University Extension Service (msstate.edu) (Accessed 6/19/23).
6. Hermel SR. Solid Footing. American Angus Association to start collecting hoof scores to generate expected progeny differences. Angus J 2015;140–1.
7. Palmer CW. Management and breeding soundness of mature bulls. Vet Clin Food Anim 2016;32:479–95.

8. Barth AD, Waldner CL. Factors affecting breeding soundness classification of beef bulls examined at the Western College of Veterinary Medicine. Can Vet J 2002;43:274–84.

9. Holyrod RG, Doogan VJ, De Faveri J, et al. Bull selection and use in northern Australia: 4. Calf output and predictors of fertility of bulls in multiple-sire herds. Anim Reprod Sci 2002;15:67–79.

10. Siqueira JB, Oba E, Pinho RO, et al. Testicular shape and andrological aspects of young Nellore bulls under extensive farming. Rev Bras Zootec 2012;41:612–7.

11. McGowan MR, Bertram JD, Fordyce G, et al. Bull selection and use in northern Australia 1.Physical traits. Anim Reprod Sci 2002;71:25–37.

12. Bonsma J., Selecting Livestock for functional efficiency, In: Myers L., Man *Must Measure: Livestock Production by Jan Bonsma*, 3rd edition, 2012, Applied Genetics Publishing, Cody, Wyoming, 47–76.

13. Durbin HJ, Lu D, Yampara-Iquise H, et al. Development of a genetic evaluation for hair shedding in American Angus cattle to improve thermotolerance. Genet Sel Evol 2020;52:63.

# The Bull Breeding Soundness Examination and Its Application in the Production Setting

E. Heath King, DVM, MS[a], Richard M. Hopper, DVM[b],*

## KEYWORDS

- Bull • Soundness • BSE • Sperm morphology • Production systems

## KEY POINTS

- It is critically important that the procedure is performed in a consistent and thorough manner.
- A breeding soundness examination (BSE) is the baseline for a diagnostic work-up in a bull suspected of infertility.
- The value of this procedure to the end user of the bull goes beyond simply establishing a prognosis for fertility.
- A BSE can be used as an aid in bull stocking strategies.

## INTRODUCTION

The breeding soundness examination (BSE) for bulls is possibly one of the most extensively described procedures in veterinary literature focused on bovine reproduction, theriogenology, or production medicine in cattle. Although the value of this procedure is well accepted by cattlemen and promoted by veterinarians and animal science extension personnel, consistency in the manner it is performed remains to be problematic. When the procedure is performed before sale inherent conflict exists because the results of the examination can negatively affect the sale and utilization for diagnostic reasons implies that a deleterious reproductive event has already occurred. The greatest value, the application of the most stringent assessment, and the potential for expanded utilization of results occur when performed for the end user.

[a] Theriogenology, Department of Pathobiology and Population Medicine, College of Veterinary Medicine, Mississippi State University, 240 Wise Center Drive, Mississippi State, MS 39762, USA; [b] Department of Clinical Sciences, College of Veterinary Medicine, Auburn University, Auburn, AL, USA
* Corresponding author. 2254 Potomac Court, Auburn, AL 36830.
*E-mail address:* richardhopperdvm@gmail.com

Vet Clin Food Anim 40 (2024) 19–27
https://doi.org/10.1016/j.cvfa.2023.08.001
0749-0720/24/© 2023 Published by Elsevier Inc.
vetfood.theclinics.com

## CHALLENGES THAT AFFECT CONSISTENCY OR VALIDITY OF RESULTS

Recently, Norman reviewed the different BSE standards in various cattle-producing countries.[1] He found that the criteria were similar with regard to evaluation of the most critical aspects, those being physical examination, reproductive tract examination, and the importance of sperm morphology. Therefore, although the different schemes are consistent in their approach, it is inconsistency in the practitioner's performance of the examination that creates discrepancies. The evaluation of a semen sample for gross motility only is paramount to not evaluating the semen, as motility is the least important metric used when evaluating a bull's potential fertility[2] compared with morphology and physical defects that might render him unable to service cattle. Additionally, while evaluation of sperm morphology is the single most important diagnostic indicator, semen with excellent sperm morphology is worthless if the bull cannot physically breed a cow. Thus, one cannot omit thorough physical and reproductive system examinations. A BSE performed by a veterinarian that conscientiously follows the standards set forth by the Society for Theriogenology (SFT)[3] avoids this issue. Additionally, the form developed by the SFT and available for use by its members is prescriptive and thus facilitates the consistent application of a BSE if used and followed. With respect to sperm evaluation, an Eosin-Nigrosin (E-N) stain is recommended, but osmolarity can be a problem. The hypo-osmolarity of the stain can cause sperm with intact plasma membranes to swell causing the sperm tail to bend artifactually. This problem is suspected when a high percentage of distal midpiece reflex defects are observed without the presence of distal droplet. Likewise, microscope quality or type is important.[4] Utilization of a scrotal circumference (SC) tape developed by Barth and others (the Reliabull; **Fig. 1**) seems to overcome discrepancies in scrotal measurements among individuals.

Bulls examined before production sales represent the greatest area for concern with respect to validity. Perhaps due to the high input costs relating to bull raising and development, owners have a strong incentive to select an individual that will "pass" all or at least an overwhelming majority of bulls presented for examination. Further complicating the question of examination validity and composition is the suggested sales term used by some breed associations. For example, the term "fertility examination" is sometimes substituted for BSE. Additionally, the examination itself, even when referred to as a BSE, can be performed by a "reproductive technician" without the oversight of a veterinarian. Regardless of one's viewpoint with regard to this issue, the authors are comfortable making the blanket statement that producers purchasing bulls at sales are generally well served by the practice of having them examined within 30 days or purchase by a veterinarian that adheres to the standards set forth by the SFT.

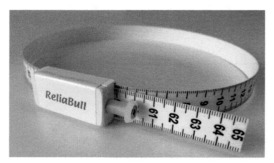

**Fig. 1.** Reliabull scrotal tape. (Reliabull™ scrotal tape. Designed by Dr. Albert Barth, Professor Emeritus in Large Animal Clinical Sciences at the University of Saskatchewan.)

## SCHEDULING THE PROCEDURE IN THE CONTEXT OF BREEDING SEASON MANAGEMENT

Although the timing for this procedure within the context of production management would seem to be intuitive, it is still useful to include this in our discussion. The authors typically recommend that a BSE be performed 30 to 60 days before turnout. This timeline allows opportunity to obtain a replacement bull if needed or for the treatment and convalescence of most hoof-related lameness, minor illness, or marginal body condition related to nutrition or parasitism. With respect to environmental conditions (extreme heat or cold) that influence the results, an argument can be made that the fluctuations in ambient temperature also occur during the breeding season and the desirable bull is one that meets the BSE standards regardless. When bulls are used for 2 breeding seasons per year, it is recommended that a BSE is performed before each.

## REVIEW OF THE BREEDING SOUNDNESS EXAMINATION
### The Physical Examination

A crucial aspect of the BSE is the determination of a bull's physical ability to thrive in a pasture or range environment as well as identify and service estrual females. Thus, a basic physical examination is performed with that goal in mind. Observing the bull as he leaves the trailer or as he moves with a group toward the holding pen provides an easy way to assess not only locomotion, potential lameness, and awareness of surroundings, but also temperament. Once restrained in the chute, confirm his identity, look at him from the front assessing facial symmetry and inspect the eyes for corneal opacity or signs of squamous carcinoma or pinkeye. Next, evaluate his body condition and if possible obtain a weight. Then carefully look at his feet and legs, specifically toe length, any curvature of the toes (screw claw), interdigital fibroma, laminitis, and swelling or joint effusion of the hock. Excessive toe length is a potential risk factor for lameness as it has been reported that dairy cattle with shorter toes and a greater dorsal hoof angle experience less hoof-related lameness throughout their lives.[5] Screw claw is considered a heritable condition[6] whether the heritability is of a primary nature or secondary due to base narrow conformation (Dr Dwight Wolfe-personal communication). A video describing how to score hooves in cattle can be found at https://www.youtube.com/watch?v=Ocplm_IGEt8. Undesirable hock conformation may result from over feeding bulls during development, natural phenotype, or a combination of both (see Chapter 2: Physical Evaluation of the Breeding Bull). The conformation of the sheath should also evaluated at this time (see Chapters 2 and 4: Medical and Surgical Management of Conditions of the Penis and Prepuce).

### The Reproductive Tract Examination

Evaluation of the external reproductive structures can be performed while measuring the SC (**Box 1**, **Fig. 2**).

The normal shape of the scrotum is pear shaped with a distinctive neck. Realize, however, that during cold weather the testes will be pulled closely to the body, altering the scrotal shape. The testes should be approximately equal size, firm when palpated, and similar to the consistency of an almost ripe orange. Testes that feel soft suggest testicular degeneration and histology images of this condition displaying extensive vacuolization illustrate this loss of density (**Fig. 3**). Conversely, hardness is likely due to fibrosis. An ultrasonic evaluation of the testes is a useful tool (**Fig. 4**) but the results of which should always be interpreted in the context of sperm morphology.[7] The testes should also move freely within the scrotum and the tail and as much of the

---

**Box 1**
**Minimum acceptable scrotal circumference values by age in months**

30 cm at less than 15 months

31 cm at greater than 15 to ≤18 months

32 cm at greater than 18 to ≤21 months

33 cm at greater than 21 to ≤24 months

34 cm at greater than 24 months

---

body and head of each epididymis as possible should be palpated. Occasionally, an epididymis will be positioned laterally, leading to a suspicion that the testicle might be partially twisted (testicular torsion). The authors have repeatedly encountered this condition and believe it is simply a variation of normal and in our experience does not seem to have a deleterious effect on fertility.

A per-rectum examination is then performed. Following introduction of your hand at about wrist level, the *urethralis muscle* can be palpated ventrally. This usually stimulates a muscular response and if not, digital pressure should be applied, as this response is useful in preparing the bull for collection via electro-ejaculation (EE). As you proceed cranially, you will encounter the prostate, which feels similar to a wedding band over your finger. Continuing forward, the paired lobular vesicular glands are encountered. Size of the vesicular glands are variable depending on the age of the bull, but they should be comparable to each other in size and consistency. The

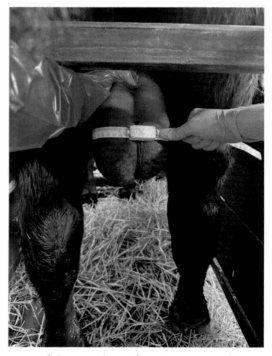

**Fig. 2.** Correct placement of the scrotal tape for an accurate and repeatable measurement.

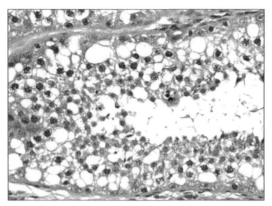

**Fig. 3.** Histology image of the testis of a bull with only 9% morphologically normal sperm. Note the pervasive vacuolization and lack of normal testicular parenchyma. Additionally, this illustrates why the testicles of bulls such as this are soft on palpation.

exhibition of pain on palpation and/or size disproportion are signs of vesicular adenitis. The paired ampullae are medial to the vesicular gland, about 1 cm in diameter, and rarely implicated with pathology. The inguinal rings are not reproductive structures, but should be identified and evaluated for current or potential herniation. This completes the examination, but to further facilitate collection, the authors advocate digital stimulation of the *urethralis muscle* followed by closing of one's hand and forward–backward movement of the arm within the rectum. The later has the purpose of "fatiguing" the rectum, which is useful in that the probe is more easily inserted.

The lubricated electro-ejaculator probe is inserted rectally and stimulation is begun. EE should result in full extension of the penis allowing for visualization and palpation if needed. Specific conditions to look for include persistent frenulum, warts, hair rings, and lacerations or fibrosis from old injuries and wounds. These can be observed on

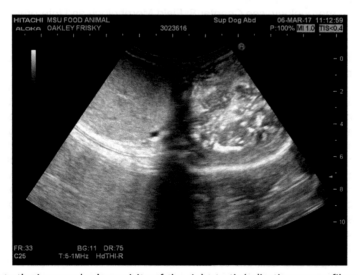

**Fig. 4.** Note the increased echogenicity of the right testis indicating severe fibrosis.

prepuce or the free portion of the penis. "Blushing" of the free portion of the penis, quickly followed by loss of erection may be visualized when there is a shunt of the corpus cavernosum. Additionally, the prepuce is evaluated for excessive/redundant tissue, which is a predisposing factor for injury. If extension of the penis does not occur during EE, it should be extended manually. Providing cranially directed pressure to the caudal aspect of the sigmoid flexure best facilitates this. If necessary, grasp the free, exposed portion of the penis with gauze to provide traction for full extension. Regardless, full visualization of the extended penis should occur.

### Evaluation of Semen

This actually begins during collection. It is best to not collect the first (all clear and even the first cloudy) emissions for evaluation. In general the color of semen grossly, watery to that of thick cream correlates with sperm concentration. Additionally, while urine contamination is possible when semen has a yellow appearance, this colorization is often the result of riboflavin pigments secreted by the ampullae and vesicular glands. A semen sample obtained near the end of the collection process that has the appearance of heavy cream, whether white or yellow in appearance is typically of diagnostic use. Following collection, handle the sample carefully to avoid cold shock and place a drop on a warmed slide and evaluate on low (40X or 100X) power. A sample suspected of urine contamination, will have poor-or-no motility (confirmation of the presence of urine can be verified with a BUN stick). The presence of the often described rapid swirls indicates that motility is adequate, as the minimal standard for individual motility is only 30%. As gross motility does not correlate well to individual progressive motility and is impacted by concentration, one is advised to evaluate a diluted (sodium citrate is better than saline) sample under a coverslip. To prepare a slide for examination of morphology, a drop of E-N stain is placed on a warm, clean slide and then mixed with a drop of semen. The resultant drop is then pushed with another slide in the same way a blood smear is done. Once dried, the slide is examined at 1000x (oil immersion) and a total of 100 sperm are counted, differentiating them as normal or having head, midpiece, or tail abnormalities. Samples that have 70% normal sperm meet the SFT standard. However, not all sperm abnormalities are equal in significance and certain abnormalities have different prognostic significance. (For more information about sperm morphology, see Chapter 8: Field Morphology and Interpretation.)

### Utilization as a Diagnostic Tool

Occasionally, bulls are presented for suspected infertility or subfertility. In these cases, historical information is critical. Determine both the pregnancy rate and staging of pregnancy from previous season(s) as well as past breeding seasons. In addition, determine if mating has been observed and whether there has been a past or recent illness. In these cases, in addition to the standard BSE, an ultrasound evaluation of the scrotal contents and internal genitalia should be performed. The spermiogram often provides the answer and if ok (>70% morphologically normal) it has been the experience of the authors that before investing resources in further diagnostic testing of the bull (sperm chromatin, etc.), it is judicious to then evaluate the cowherd. When there are fewer than 70% normal sperm, the prevalent sperm abnormality may provide clues to the etiology or more importantly the prognosis for recovery. Although a comprehensive discussion on sperm morphology follows later (Chapter 8), a few abnormalities will be discussed here. When the proximal droplet defect seems in prevalent numbers in the middle-aged or older bull, testicular degeneration is suspected.[8] Conversely, in the young, peripubertal bull, this seems to be transient in nature and the bull can be deferred for subsequent retesting. The knobbed acrosome defect which is considered uncompensable, when prevalent in a spermiogram is significant in that it has been found that normal appearing sperm within that ejaculate may also be affected and yield reduced fertilization rates.[9] The obvious conclusion to this being that the level of subfertility exceeds the apparent level observed. Detached or "free" heads are most commonly encountered in the young peripubertal bull, but a very dense, highly concentrated sample, with poor motility and 70% to 80% detached heads, is indicative of semen stasis. Normally, sperm are continually released and exit through micturition, so stasis or sperm accumulation is abnormal and the bull will have to be collected numerous times until a potentially normal sample can be obtained. This differs from the so-called "rusty load", which is characterized by a bull that has not been breeding and has an increased percentage of abnormalities in a first collection followed by better quality semen on the subsequent collection.

## UTILIZATION IN THE PRODUCTION SETTING

The BSE performed on a bull for the owner/user facilitates a discussion between veterinarian and cowman, allowing the establishment of parameters that may vary or go beyond the SFT standards. These departures from the standards will reflect the production goals of the cattleman. For example, the seedstock producer should have a low tolerance for even slight hoof or limb conformational issues, while those might be acceptable for another producer with a bull used in a terminal cross. What level of fertility is acceptable? A producer planning on having a bull collected for semen cryopreservation so that he could synchronize and breed a large group and then use that same bull for "clean-up" would need a bull's whose morphology and motility exceeded standard percentages.

A potential value added aspect of a BSE that is routinely under-utilized, is its employment for assigning stocking rates. Research has shown that in single sire mating groups bull-to-cow ratios in excess of the often cited, 1:25, can be utilized, with no difference in pregnancy rates at 1:44 or even 1:60.[10] The caveat of course being that the bulls meet the SFT standards. Recent work providing retrospective data on bull to cow ratios used following artificial insemination occurring in conjunction with an estrus synchronization, stocking ratios up to 1:73 (actually an effective rate of 1:44 as based on cows open after AI) without deceases in pregnancy rate compared with lower stocking.[11] There are several considerations when decreasing the stocking rate of bulls to cows. First, it is crucial that bulls have the physical ability to complete the mating act and possess good libido. High libido bulls often display increased services per cow and reserve levels of sperm drop rapidly with each ejaculate (75% in the first 10 ejaculates). Therefore, bulls with SC measures greater than the minimum should be selected when expanding the bull-to-cow ratio.[12] Additionally, a short breeding season length of less than 50 days could place added pressure on a bull battery and caution should be observed before advising a producer to use fewer bulls.

When assigning the stocking rates for multi-sire breeding groups the variables of individual bull libido and the effect of social dominance are difficult to measure. Bull libido is not examined or scored on a standard BSE. Attempts to measure bull libido have been made by performing servicing capacity tests, where the number of females or mounts that a bull makes is recorded over a predetermined time-period. These tests lack standardization, and the results vary depending on the age and breed of the bulls tested.[13] Assessment of libido or willingness to mate must therefore be determined by producer observation during the breeding season. Social dominance, where a dominant bull suppresses the mating activity of others in the group, has been documented. This dominance tends to be expressed by older more senior bulls and has the greatest impact on calf output per bull when the stocking density of bulls is high.[14,15] A large 2 year study in northern Australia, utilizing *Bos indicus* bulls, investigated the impact of stocking density on social dominance and calf output per bull. They demonstrated no effect on conception patterns between groups when the stocking rate of bulls to cows was reduced from 1:17 to 1:40. Furthermore, the variation in calf output per bull and bull injury were also reduced at lower stocking rates. Overall pregnancy rates did differ between groups, but the difference was attributed to forage availability and body condition variation between groups.[15] It is important to note that the bulls used in this study and the ones sited above were all 2 years of age and older. Breeding behavior in young bulls less than 2 years of age does vary but when measured typically does improve with experience.[16]

## SUMMARY

This procedure as a prognostic indicator of fertility has a high economic value for cattle producers, but to have that value it must be performed competently and consistently. Utilization as a diagnostic tool is also of importance. An additional, but typically underutilized value for this procedure centers on its use in proscribing bull-to-cow ratios. Client education continues to be crucial.

## DISCLOSURE

The authors have nothing to disclose.

## REFERENCES

1. Norman ST. Bull breeding soundness evaluation: comparative review of different standards. In: Hopper RM, editor. Bovine reproduction. 2nd edition. Wiley; 2021.
2. Fitzpatrick LA, Fordyce G, McGowan MR, et al. Bull selection and use in northern Australia Part 2. Semen Traits. Anim Reprod Sci 2002;71:39–49.
3. Koziol JH, Armstrong CL. Society for Theriogenology Manual for Breeding Soundness Examination of Bulls, 2nd ed. 2018.
4. Freneau GE, Chenoweth PJ, Ellis R, et al. Sperm morphology of beef bulls evaluated by two different methods. Anim Reprod Sci 2010;118:176–81.
5. Vermunt JJ, Greenough PR. Structural characteristics of the bovine claw: horn growth and wear, horn hardness and claw conformation. Br Vet J 1995;151: 157–80.
6. AABP Lameness Committee. AABP Fact Sheet, An approach to corkscrew claw.
7. Barth AD. Testicular degeneration. In: Hopper RM, editor. Bovine reproduction. Wiley; 2015. p. 103–8.
8. Hopper R. Semen evaluation and overview of common sperm abnormalities. Clinical Theriogenology 2015;7:261–8.
9. Thundathil J, Palomino J, Barth AD, et al. Fertilizing characteristics of bovine sperm with flattened or indented acrosomes. Anim Reprod Sci 2001;67:231–43.
10. Rupp GP, Ball L, Shoop MC, et al. Reproductive efficiency of bulls in natural service: effects of male to female ratio and single- vs multiple-sire breeding groups. J Am Vet Med Assoc 1977;171(7):639–42.
11. Timlin CL, Dias NW, Hungerford L, et al. A retrospective analysis of bull: cow ratio effects on pregnancy rates of beef cows previously enrolled in fixed-time artificial insemination protocols. Transl Anim Sci 2021;5(3):txab129.

12. Almquist JO, Amann RP. Reproductive Capacity of Dairy Bulls. II. Gonadal and Extra-gonadal Sperm Reserves as Determined by Direct Counts and Depletion Trials; Dimensions and Weight of Genitalia. J Dairy Sci 1961;44:1668.

13. Petherick J. A review of some of the factors affecting expression of libido in beef cattle, and individual bull and herd fertility. Appl Anim Behav 2005;90:185–205.

14. Chenoweth PJ. Bull drive and reproductive behavior. In: Chenoweth PJ, editor. Topics in bull fertility. Ithaca (NY): International Veterinary Information Service; 2000. Available at: www.ivis.org.

15. Fordyce G, Fitzpatrick L, Copper N, et al. Bull selection and use in northern Australia 5. Social behavior and management. Anim Reprod Sci 2002;71:81–99.

16. Boyd GW, Lunstra DD, Corah LR. Serving capacity of crossbred yearling beef bulls. 1. Single-sire mating behavior and fertility during average and heavy mating loads at pasture. J Anim Sci 1989;67:60–71.

# Field Morphology and Interpretation

Jennifer H. Koziol, DVM, MS, DACT

## KEYWORDS

- Semen evaluation • Bulls • Sperm morphology • Spermiogram

## KEY POINTS

- Semen morphology evaluation in the field should always be performed at 1000× with oil immersion.
- Development of a spermiogram will aid the practitioner to interpret potential fertility of semen at the time of sampling as well as determine potential causes of an abnormal spermiogram.
- Bulls, which experience stress or impairment of thermoregulation of the testes for any reason, often experience a transitory decrease in the quality of sperm morphology. This can be recognized by a sequence of appearances of morphologic defects coupled with a thorough patient history.
- Nutrition either in excess or deficiency can impact sperm quality.
- Testicular degeneration occurs following insult to a testis(es). The extent of the testicular degeneration depends on the severity and duration of the testicular insult and is often transitory in nature except for in the most extreme cases.

## INTRODUCTION

Multiple studies have shown that approximately 15% to 20% of bulls at any given time point will be marked as questionable/deferred or unsatisfactory potential breeders due to either inadequate semen quality, lack of physical soundness, or both.[1-5] Morphologically abnormal sperm has long been associated with male infertility, and assessment of these abnormalities has been clearly identified as a fundamental component of analysis of semen quality.[2,6-11] Sperm morphology is an excellent predictor of the outcome of natural mating, artificial insemination, and *in vitro fertilization*,[8,12-14] and there is a relationship between morphologically abnormal bull sperm and poor DNA quality.[9] When using standards established by the Society for Theriogenology, the most common reason that bulls are classified as unsatisfactory or deferred is unacceptable sperm morphology.[1,15]

The evaluation of sperm morphology provides the veterinarian a noninvasive method to evaluate current and past testicular and epididymal function, providing

Texas Tech School of Veterinary Medicine, 7671 Evans Drive, Amarillo, TX 79106, USA
*E-mail address:* jkoziol@ttu.edu

Vet Clin Food Anim 40 (2024) 29–40
https://doi.org/10.1016/j.cvfa.2023.06.001
0749-0720/24/© 2023 Elsevier Inc. All rights reserved.

information that mimics that which can be gained by a testicular biopsy. It is important to remember that semen evaluation is a snapshot in time and on the day of collection only evaluates what the bull has spermatogenically produced in the last 61 days plus 10 days which encompasses the length of sperm transportation through the epididymis. Consequently, a bull's spermiogram can differ from evaluation to evaluation pending any disturbances in spermatogenesis. This necessitates the need for veterinarians to use patient history, clinical examination, and findings of a complete breeding soundness examination to make recommendations regarding current and future breeding potential of a bull. However, even that information may not give a complete clinical picture and if the unsatisfactory potential breeder warrants the cost; multiple semen evaluations spread 6 to 8 weeks apart may be necessary to evaluate the true future breeding potential. These facts should encourage veterinarians to make thorough notes regarding the percentages of specific types of defects noted during evaluation of the sperm morphology slide. This will allow for future evaluations to be compared with previous findings and determine if sperm morphology and testicular recovery is occurring or not.

Diligent evaluation of sperm morphology in the field setting can be easily accomplished with proper equipment and prior planning. Veterinarians should be mindful of possible environmental effects that will be encountered including wind that will cool the surface of the slide warmer, direct sunshine that may impair ability to easily visualize slides through the microscope and affect semen quality, and the myriad of other weather conditions that food animal veterinarians encounter in the field. The veterinarian and cattle producer can discuss possible ways to mitigate those effects to avoid any environmental conditions that would negatively affect the potential outcome of a bull's breeding soundness examination (BBSE). Alternatively, the veterinarian may elect to swiftly evaluate progressive motility in the field and prepare a sperm morphologic slide that is carefully identified and stored in a slide box to evaluate on return to the clinic.

### Basic Field Supplies Related to Semen Morphology Evaluation

- Quality microscope (bright-field or phase-contrast) with 100× objective
- Slide warmer
- Quality microscope slides
- Pipettes
- Eosin–nigrosin stain or tubes with fixative if utilizing phase contrast
- Microscope cover slips if using phase contrast
- Immersion oil
- Cell counter
- Pencil or permanent marker for identification of slides
- Slide box
- Kimwipes and microscope cleaning supplies

### Microscopes

Microscopic evaluation of sperm morphology is a pillar of successful sperm evaluation and breeding soundness examinations of bulls. The three basic types of light microscopy are bright-field, phase-contrast, and differential interface contrast (DIC). Most conventional microscopes have a bright-field function and many also have phase contrast capability. However, DIC is expensive and is generally restricted to use in research or andrology laboratories.

Bright-field microscopy is suitable for examination of morphology using stained semen smears. Morphology evaluations must always be performed using the oil immersion (100×) objective lens; with eyepieces of 10 to 12.5×, the total magnification is 1000 to 1250× (hereafter referred to as 1000×). Morphology evaluation at lower magnification should not be performed as it results in failure to recognize many sperm abnormalities.[16–18] In addition, mineral oil should never be used in the place of immersion oil.

Utilization of phase-contrast microscopy allows examination of unstained, coverslipped, preparations prepared by mixing semen with warmed 10% neutral buffered formalin or buffered formal saline in a sterile tube followed by an aliquot being placed on a microscope slide and cover slipped as well as slides stained with Feulgen stain.[19] The evaluation of sperm morphology using phase contrast at 1000× is preferred over the use of stained preparations by some practitioners, as defects such as nuclear vacuoles,[20] acrosomal defects, and abnormal DNA in the case of Feulgen-stained slides are easier to identify. However, these defects can also readily be identified with high-quality bright-field microscopes.

An anecdotal litmus test to determine the quality of a microscope that one is using is the ability of an evaluator to easily identify diadem defects with either their bright-field or phase-contrast microscope(s). Diadem defects are considered the most commonly missed defect.[16–18] If an evaluator does not visualize a diadem defect during the full length of their BBSE season they should consider if their microscope is of high enough quality.

Cleaning of microscopes is of upmost importance to keep them in good working order. Professional microscope cleaning services can be set up on a routine basis pending the amount of field use or in-house cleaning can be performed. Camera cleaning tools are often useful in the cleaning process. Kimwipes and lens cleaner should be kept in the microscope case to clean objectives following end of day as immersion oil should not be left on objectives. It is also useful to quickly clean any objectives that are inadvertently dragged through immersion oil or become soiled during field work.

### Other Equipment

Slide warmers are not only critical for proper evaluation of sperm motility as they aid in preventing cold shock but also proper preparation of sperm morphology slides. Slide warmers should be used to keep all glassware (slides and coverslips) and pipettes that will encounter semen post-collection at a temperature sufficient as not to introduce cold shock. Typically set at 98°F/37°C, the slide warmer is crucial for making sure that slides prepared with eosin–nigrosin dry quickly. The slide warmer can also be used to keep fixative for phase-contrast warm as not to induce cold shock before fixation. Consequences of slow drying are discussed in detail below in the section outlining morphologic abnormalities caused by iatrogenic means. Slide warmers are equally important when using phase contrast as not to induce cold shock in semen before fixation in the preservative.

High-quality microscope slides and coverslips should be purchased for evaluation of sperm morphology. As morphology slides are examined at 1000×, any unevenness in the surface of the slide or coverslip can create difficulty when trying to streak out stained slides or focus and maintain focus at 1000× high magnification. It is also important to make sure that slides and coverslips free of fingerprints along with detergent free as this can cause abnormalities in the staining or fixing process.

### Preparing Sperm Morphology Slides

Slide preparation is crucial for proper evaluation of sperm morphology and requires practice and attention to detail. Common errors include too many sperm per slide

(**Fig. 1**); slides stained too dark or too light; and slow drying resulting in cracks and stain artifacts. There are multiple ways to create stained slides. Some may prefer to streak out slides using another glass slide in a manner similar to producing a blood smear (**Fig. 2**), whereas others prefer to use a wood applicator stick to roll the sample out. Some practitioners believe that the wood applicator stick results in less mechanical damage to the sperm (detached heads, damaged acrosomes). However, no studies support this clinical suspicion. Slides can be viewed anywhere along the length but usually half way down the slide is a good place to start as the cells are usually evenly distributed with good background stain. However, there is limited evidence that an evaluator should count cells throughout a large portion of the slide to allow for a fair assessment of the bull. Reading in a small section of the slide may lead to false conclusions regarding the potential breeding status of that animal.[20]

Wet mounts can be made for evaluation of sperm morphology by phase-contrast microscopy at 1000×. Freshly ejaculated semen must be diluted, and motility completely stopped to allow for accurate evaluate. This can be accomplished with the addition of 0.2% glutaraldehyde in phosphate-buffered saline, buffered formal saline, or with neutral buffered formalin. Buffered formal saline is often preferred as glutaraldehyde and neutral buffered formalin lead to clumping of sperm cells making evaluation of cells extremely cumbersome. To prepare a wet mount slide, a 2 to 3 mm drop of diluted semen is placed on a warm clean microscope slide with a pipette. The author prefers graduated tip pipettes as to better control the size of the drop. Following placement of the drop, a cover slip is placed over top. Allow the drop to evenly distribute under the coverslip before placing a drop of oil on the coverslip for examination at 1000×. Slides should be allowed to sit upward of 15 minutes to allow semen to settle into a single layer before observation to prevent sperm cells from laying in multiple planes and consequently creating the artifact of misshapen or narrow based heads.[21,22] The preparation should be also very thin to avoid sperm laying on their edges rather than flat. Wet mount slides can be viewed at any location along the coverslip with the exception of near the edges as this is where a higher number of dead cells tend to accumulate.[8]

### Evaluation of Sperm Morphology Slides

Live/dead stains, also referred to as supravital stains, such as eosin–nigrosin and eosin–aniline blue, are commonly used for routine morphologic examination of sperm

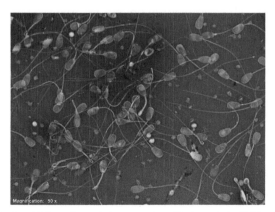

**Fig. 1.** Sperm cells should be adequately spaced so that each individual cell can be thoroughly examined. This slide is too crowded impeding proper evaluation.

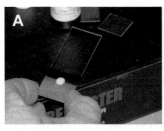 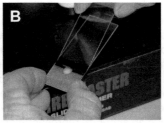 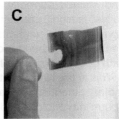

**Fig. 2.** Preparation of eosin–nigrosin stained slide. (*A*) A line of eosin-nigrosin stain is placed followed by a small drop of semen above the stain. (*B*) A second slide is taken and held at a 30 - degree angle. the slide is settled into the stain backed into the semen rocked back and forth to allow even distribution of the semen and stain on the leading age and then streaked out. (*C*) The slide should have a even look and should not be excessively light or dark.

in the field due to ease of making slides and the ability for the practitioner to quickly read once the stain has dried. Drying occurs in seconds with the aid of slide warmers set at the appropriate temperature.[23] In a study by Tanghe and colleagues, eosin–nigrosin staining of sperm was the only bull sperm quality parameter evaluated that demonstrated a significant association with pronucleus formation in vitro fertilization.[24] When using live/dead stains, nigrosin or aniline blue provide a background, whereas eosin acts as a vital stain. Functional plasma membranes of viable sperm prevent penetration of eosin into the cell; therefore, viable sperm appear white. In contrast, eosin penetrates damaged cell membranes, staining injured or nonviable sperm pink.

Partially stained sperm, with a pink posterior portion and a white anterior portion of the sperm head, are sometimes observed. These sperm have suffered membrane damage, yet the acrosome remained intact. This staining pattern occurs because the acrosomal membrane is tightly adhered to the nucleus at the equatorial region and penetration of the eosin stain under the acrosome is initially impeded at the equatorial region.[16] Partially stained sperm are more common when semen samples are processed under less than ideal conditions, suggesting that sperm membrane damage or cell death occurred very recently (**Fig. 3**).

When assessing the proportion of sperm staining alive, it may be relevant to only count sperm stained completely white. When semen has been handled properly

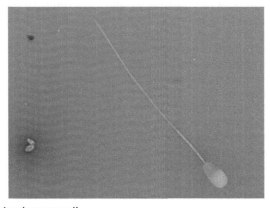

**Fig. 3.** Partially stained sperm cell.

and stained correctly, the percentage excluding eosin, and therefore considered "alive" is highly correlated to progressive motility. The percentage alive is also highly correlated the percentage of morphologically normal. This suggests that when is semen handled under optimal or near-optimal conditions, a high proportion of bulls with good sperm morphology will also have good sperm motility.[2]

This is not to suggest that adequate motility is sufficient for deeming a bull a satisfactory potential breeder or only "alive" cells should be counted during evaluation of a sperm morphology slide; a minimum of 100 cells should be counted regardless of dead or alive status to give an accurate representation of the current state of the ejaculate. The accuracy of the assessment of marginal bulls can be improved by counting 300 to 500 cells.

The goal for examining sperm morphology is to determine the percentage and types of sperm abnormalities present in a sample and thereby construct a spermiogram (description of sperm morphology). The spermiogram may be used to interpret potential fertility of semen at the time of sampling as well as determine potential causes of an abnormal spermiogram. Knowledge of probable causes of abnormalities coupled with timeline of occurrence of abnormal morphology following a testicular insult of any kind may allow the practitioner to develop a prognosis for recovery. Veterinarians can accordingly aid their client in making an informed decision regarding future directions about a bull in question.[16,18]

Determination of a spermiogram is facilitated using a differential cell counter. Mechanical cell counters often allow evaluators to press 2 or more keys simultaneously to record more than one defect within the same sperm while counting the individual sperm only once. With this system, a more accurate spermiogram may be produced. If this system is used it will be important to communicate such to owners that the total number may exceed 100 and if evaluating sell bulls a note should be provided on any breeding soundness evaluation sheets that will accompany the bull on purchase.

When sperm morphology is good, differential counting of 100 sperm is adequate to determine a spermiogram. However, when the percentage of abnormal sperm present is high, counting at least 300 sperm may be necessary to produce an accurate spermiogram.

### Interpretation of the Morphology

Spermiograms are defined as a description of sperm morphology during evaluation. An abnormal spermiogram with supporting evidence from the history and physical examination can give insights into reasons for abnormal testicular function and consequently allow formation of a prognosis for recovery or potential treatment. When an abnormal spermiogram is found, the types and number of abnormalities combined with history regarding environment, nutrition, and health status can be used to compile a reason for spermiogram disturbances noted. The veterinarian can then use that information to make a diagnosis and prognosis for recovery.

The most common causes of abnormal spermatogenesis in males include: abnormal testicular thermoregulation; hormonal imbalances, particularly those associated with stress; and effect(s) of toxins or expression of deleterious genes.[25] Stress typically elevates systemic cortisol concentrations, profoundly decreasing release of luteinizing hormone (LH) and testosterone.[26–28] Stress has many origins, including environment, illness, nutrition, or injury, causing changes in the spermiogram similar to those induced by disruption of thermoregulation. The primary spermatocyte is extremely sensitive to alterations in the hormonal milieu secondary to stress or illness. For example, in cases of testicular degeneration, the changes appear first in the cytoplasm, centrosomes, and spindles at the level of the primary spermatocyte which predispose to disturbances in the developing spermatid.[8,29]

A testicular insult of sufficient duration (>48 hours) may result in disruption of critical maturation processes for spermatids, and recently released spermatozoa in the testes and epididymis leading to the appearance of certain morphologic abnormalities such as proximal droplets and distal midpiece reflexes (DMRs) in the spermiogram.[8,16,25] Mild disturbances may only affect spermatids or epididymal spermatozoa with a short-lived period of increased numbers of morphologic abnormalities. A study characterizing the sequential appearance of morphologic abnormalities noted that there were differences between animals in the overall degree of response to the negative stimulus reflected in the proportion of morphologically abnormal sperm and the proportion of certain types of defects.[25] More severe or prolonged disturbances cause destruction of the spermatocytes and spermatogonia. Not all seminiferous tubules will be affected the same which accounts for the diverse population of sperm defects that may be noted on evaluation. The author discusses some common reasons for abnormal spermiograms as follows.

## Immaturity

Immaturity is often recognized in the spermiogram by the observation of a high numbers of immature sperm cells also known as spheroids combined with high levels of sperm with proximal droplets and distal droplets. Peripubertal bulls often have a high percentage of sperm with proximal droplets in the ejaculate.[8,30–34] As bulls mature, the number of proximal droplets in the spermiogram should decrease.[8]

Immature sperm cells are quite variable in size, depending on whether the cell is a primary or a secondary spermatocyte or a spermatid.[35,36] Immature sperm cells must be differentiated from white blood cells in semen. This differentiation can be accomplished by staining a dried semen smear in Diff-quik, new methylene blue, or Wright's giemsa. Once the stain is dried the round cells can be evaluated and a final diagnosis of immature sperm cell or white blood cell can be made by the evaluator.

If a diagnosis of immaturity is made the bull should be reevaluated in 4 to 6 weeks to allow for maturation. It is unwise to speculate on the future breeding potential of a yearling bull (12–15 months of age). A review of records found that only 35% of physically normal yearling bulls which were declared decision deferred on the first examination went on to pass subsequent breeding soundness examinations.[16]

## Stress

Stress for any reason (environment, nutrition, social, illness, injury, and so forth) causes a rise in cortisol which has negative feedback to the hypothalamus and pituitary causing a decrease in follicle stimulating hormone (FSH), luteining hormone (LH), and testosterone. This leads to sperm changes not only in the testes but also epididymis. The most notable defect and the first morphologic defect to be noted following a stress event is the DMR. DMR defects are due to an abnormal hormonal milieu most notably a decrease in testosterone levels in the cauda epididymis, specifically, the distal third of the cauda epididymis.[8] High concentrations of testosterone are necessary for normal epididymal function.[37]

Although DMRs are the most characteristic change, you may notice a variety of defects can be found following a stressful event including proximal droplets, detached heads and mitochondrial disturbances, knobbed acrosomes, nuclear vacuoles, coiled principal pieces, and pyriform heads. **Fig. 4** depicts the normal progression of abnormal sperm morphology following an acute period of stress.

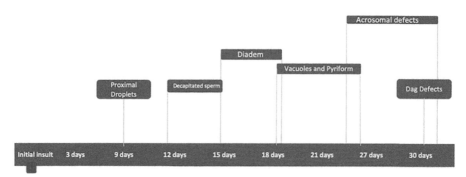

**Fig. 4.** Normal progression of abnormal sperm morphology following an acute period of stress.

## Nutrition

Testis mass and consequent spermatogenesis fluctuates based on metabolic cues, and appropriate nutritional management remains important throughout life.[18] Excessive body fat is unfavorable for bulls as deposition of fat in the scrotum reduces the ability of the testes to appropriately thermoregulate resulting in poor semen quality and resulting in testicular degeneration.[38] In the other extreme, insufficient nutrition may result in stress and reduced semen quality. Bull batteries that have inadequate nutrition especially in the winter or times of extreme drought have been shown to reduce number of bulls with satisfactory semen quality at the time of BBSE.[2,39]

Young bulls transitioning from high-grain diets to pasture or low-energy diet following sales can create significant stress for the animal. This can be compounded if the young bull also encounters social dominance or hierarchical challenges.[40] Proper nutritional management of young bulls before, during, and after their first breeding seasons is critical to maintaining the longevity of bulls in the herd. Bulls should be maintained on a diet with adequate amounts of balanced dietary protein and energy sources to ensure proper endocrine development to support spermatogenesis.[18] Vitamin A deficiency has deleterious effects on germinal cell populations, resulting in loss of all cells in seminiferous tubules other than spermatogonia and Sertoli cells. There is minimal evidence that deficiencies of B vitamins, vitamin C, D, or E, calcium, manganese, zinc, iodine, potassium, or selenium directly cause bull infertility.[5] Deficiencies of cobalt, iron, zinc, and copper may be associated with anemia, lack of appetite, and weight loss, thereby having negative effects on male reproduction.[5] Copper deficiency reportedly must be severe to affect spermatogenesis.

## Testicular Degeneration/Regeneration

Testicular degeneration occurs following an insult to the testicle. Potential insults include trauma, stress, abnormal testicular thermoregulation, toxins, ischemia, nutritional deficiencies or excess, infection, sperm outflow obstructions, and neoplasia. Testicular degeneration in the bull may present as a unilateral or bilateral condition and may be permanent but is most often temporary. The extent of the testicular degeneration depends on the severity and duration of the testicular insult. Alterations in the hormonal milieu within the testicle as discussed above affect the seminiferous tubules. In severe cases, seminiferous tubules may be severely damaged and slough differentiated cells into the tubular lumen. When empty tubules in the testes lose turgidity the testes become noticeably softer, and the change is recognized as testicular degeneration.[41]

The appearance of teratozoospermia is commonly observed in cases of testicular degeneration. No single morphologic aberration is exclusive to degeneration. Small numbers of spheroids, which are believed to be immature spermatogenic cells, may be seen as well as teratoid forms and medusa cells. DMRs, proximal cytoplasmic droplets, Dag-like and other midpiece disruptions, coiled principal pieces, detached heads, tapered and pyriform heads, knobbed acrosomes, all types of nuclear vacuoles, microcephalic sperm, and sperm with abnormal DNA condensation were evident following known insults to spermatogenesis.[16,25] The degree of damage to the seminiferous tubules determines the time period to recover. It may take repetitive spermiogram analysis to determine where in the stages of degeneration or regeneration the bull is currently at.

## Toxins

Many toxins have potential to affect spermatogenesis, although few naturally occurring cases have been documented.[5] Gossypol, a phenolic toxin in the pigment glands of cottonseed, impairs sperm production in several species, including ruminants. Free gossypol in cottonseed and cottonseed meal can disrupt spermatogenesis, leading to increased numbers of morphologically abnormal sperm and decreased sperm motility. Bulls fed diets containing free gossypol at levels as low as 8 mg/kg per day for 56 days produced increased numbers of sperm with segmental aplasia of the mitochondrial sheath and other midpiece defects, proximal droplets, strongly folded or coiled tails, tailless (detached) heads, simple bent, and terminally coiled tails (coiled principal pieces).[42–44] Production of defective sperm induced by gossypol exposure is reversible within 28 days after removal of gossypol from the diet.

Producers and veterinarians are often concerned about potential effects of therapeutic agents on semen quality. Exogenous corticosteroids (eg, dexamethasone) depress pituitary gonadotrophin secretions and can adversely affect spermatogenesis.[25] In contrast, several commonly used antibiotics including tilmicosin, oxytetracycline, dihydrostreptomycin, and the anti-inflammatory agent phenylbutazone had no adverse effects on semen quality.[5]

## Genetic Predisposition

Although adverse environmental influences are the most common cause of abnormal spermatogenesis, an increasing number of sperm defects are recognized as having a genetic origin.[45] A table of sperm defects that have known genetic modes of transmission are listed below. One should have suspicions of a genetic influence when a high proportion of the ejaculate is affected by the same morphologic abnormality with minimal other morphologic abnormalities in the ejaculate (**Table 1**).

## Iatrogenic Changes

Iatrogenic changes noted in the spermiogram are mostly associated with slide preparation. The most common change noted are those due to hypoosmotic changes whether that comes from stain, prolonged drying times, cold slides, or cold shock of ejaculate before staining. Hypoosmotic changes are of high suspicion when there is a high percentage of bent midpieces. Characteristically, these midpieces have no retained droplet within the bend which aids in differentiating this iatrogenic defect from DMRs. Other iatrogenic defects that may be noted are high numbers of detached heads from excessive pressure during the slide making process and cracking of the stain due to prolonged drying times which can create the appearance of artificial defects of the acrosome.

| Table 1 Heritable Morphological Abnormalities in Bovine Sperm | |
|---|---|
| Acrosome defects | 1. Knobbed acrosomes |
| | 2. Ruffled, incomplete acrosomes |
| Head defects | 1. Abnormal DNA condensation |
| | 2. Decapitated sperm defect |
| | 3. Round head |
| | 4. Rolled head |
| | 5. Nuclear crest |
| Midpiece abnormalities | 1. Dag defect |
| | 2. Corkscrew defect |
| | 3. Pseudodroplet |
| Tail defects | 1. Tail stump defect |
| | 2. Primary ciliary dyskinesia |

## SUMMARY

A proper evaluation of semen morphology during a BBSE is crucial to determining the potential breeding status of a bull. The evaluation of sperm morphology can give the practitioner invaluable insight into the function of the testis and epididymis and in the case of poor sperm production potential reasons for the defects being seen and a timeline of when the testicular insult occurred. This interpretation assists the veterinarian and bull owner in making decisions regarding the fate of the bull and future breeding management options. BBSE is one of the most economically sound investments that a cow–calf producer can make regarding herd profitability and it is our job as a veterinarian to perform our examination with knowledge and integrity.

## CLINICS CARE POINTS

- The spermatogenic cylce is bulls is 61 days.
- Semen morphology should always be evaluated at 1000X with oil immersion to identify all defects present.
- Following an acute stressful even DMRs can be noted int the semen as soon as 3-5 days after the event.

## REFERENCES

1. Carson RL, Koziol JH, Wenzel JGW, et al. Twenty year trends of bull breeding sounndness examinations at a teaching hospital. Clin Therio 2014;6:495–501.
2. Barth AD, Waldner CL. Factors affecting breeding soundness classification of beef bulls examined at the Western College of Veterinary Medicine. Can Vet J 2002;43:274–84.
3. Carroll E, Ball L, Scott JA. Breeding soundness in bulls - a summary of 10,940 examinations. J AmVet Med Assoc 1963;142:1105–11.
4. Elmore RG, Bierschwal CJ, Martin CE, et al. A summary of 1127 breeding soundness examinations in beef bulls. Theriogenology 1975;3:209–18.
5. Kennedy SP, Spitzer JC, Hopkins FM, et al. Breeding soundness evaluations of 3,648 yearling beef bulls using the 1993 Society for Theriogenology guidelines. Theriogenology 2002;58:947–61.

6. Kubo-Irie M, Matsumiya K, Iwamoto T, et al. Morphological abnormalities in the spermatozoa of fertile and infertile men. Mol Reprod Dev 2005;70:70–81.
7. Ostermeier GC, Sargeant GA, Yandell BS, et al. Relationship of bull fertility to sperm nuclear shape. J Androl 2001;22:595–603.
8. Barth AD, Oko RJ. Abnomal morphology of bovine spermatozoa. Malden: Blackwell Publishing Inc; 1989.
9. Enciso M, Cisale H, Johnston SD, et al. Major morphological sperm abnormalities in the bull are related to sperm DNA damage. Theriogenology 2011;76:23–32.
10. Parkinson TJ. Evaluation of fertility and infertility in natural service bulls. Vet J 2004;168:215–29.
11. Kastelic JP, Thundathil JC. Breeding soundness evaluation and semen analysis for predicting bull fertility. Reprod Domest Anim 2008;43:368–73.
12. Wiltbank J, Parish N. Pregnancy rate in cows and heifers bred to bulls selected for semen quality. Theriogenology 1986;25:779–83.
13. Saacke R, Dalton J, Nadir S, et al. Relationship of seminal traits and insemination time to fertilization rate and embryo quality. Anim Reprod Sci 2000;60:663–77.
14. Söderquist L, Janson L, Larsson K, et al. Sperm morphology and fertility in AI bulls. Transbound Emerg Dis 1991;38:534–43.
15. Carson RL, Wenzel JG. Observations using the new bull-breeding soundness evaluation forms in adult and young bulls. Vet Clin North Am Food Anim Pract 1997;13:305–11.
16. Barth AD. Bull breeding soundness. 3rd ed. Saskatoon: Western Canadian Association of Bovine Practitioners; 2013.
17. Koziol JH, Armstrong CL. Sperm morphology of domestic animals. Hoboken: John Wiley & Sons; 2022.
18. Koziol JH, Armstrong CL. Society for Theriogenology manual for breeding soundness examination of bulls. 2nd ed. Montgomery: Society for Theriogenology; 2018.
19. Sekoni V, Gustafsson B, Mather E. Influence of wet fixation, staining techniques, and storage time on bull sperm morphology. Nord Vet Med 1980;33:161–6.
20. Menon AG, Thundathil JC, Wilde R, et al. Validating the assessment of bull sperm morphology by veterinary practitioners. Can Vet J 2011;52:407.
21. Barth AD, Bowman PA, Bo GA, et al. Effect of narrow sperm head shape on fertility in cattle. Can Vet J 1992;33:31–9.
22. Thundathil J, Palasz AT, Mapletoft RJ, et al. An investigation of the fertilizing characteristics of pyriform-shaped bovine spermatozoa. Anim Reprod Sci 1999;57: 35–50.
23. Hancock J. A staining technique for the study of temperature-shock in semen. Nature 1951;167:323–4.
24. Tanghe S, Van Soom A, Sterckx V, et al. Assessment of different sperm quality parameters to predict in vitro fertility of bulls. Reprod Domest Anim 2002;37: 127–32.
25. Barth AD, Bowman PA. The sequential appearance of sperm abnormalities after scrotal insulation or dexamethasone treatment in bulls. Can Vet J 1994;35: 93–102.
26. Welsh T, McCraw R, Johnson B. Influence of corticosteroids on testosterone production in the bull. Biol Reprod 1979;21:755–63.
27. Welsh T, Randel R, Johnson B. Temporal relationships among peripheral blood concentrations of corticosteroids, luteinizing hormone and testosterone in bulls. Theriogenology 1979;12:169–79.

28. Welsh TH Jr, Johnson BH. Stress-induced alterations in secretion of corticosteroids, progesterone, luteinizing hormone, and testosterone in bulls. Endocrinology 1981;109:185–90.
29. Knudsen O. Cytomorphological investigations into the spermiocytogenesis of bulls with normal fertility and bulls with acquired disturbances in spermiogenesis. Acta Pathol Microbiol Scand Suppl 1954;101:1–79.
30. Johnson KR, Dewey CE, Bobo JK, et al. Prevalence of morphologic defects in spermatozoa from beef bulls. J Am Vet Med Assoc 1998;213:1468–71.
31. Lagerlöf N. Morphological studies on the change in sperm structure and in the testes of bulls with decreased or abolished fertility. Acta Pathol Microbiol Scand 1934;19:254–66.
32. Ruttle J, Ezaz Z, Sceery E. Some factors influencing semen characteristics in range bulls. J Anim Sci 1975;41:1069–76.
33. Saacke R. Morphology of the sperm and its relationship to fertility. Proc 3$^{rd}$ Tech Conf AI Reprod 1970;17–30.
34. Smith MF, Morris DL, Amoss MS, et al. Relationships among fertility, scrotal circumference, seminal quality, and libido in Santa Gertrudis bulls. Theriogenology 1981;16:379–97.
35. Swerczek T. Immature germ cells in the semen of thoroughbred stallions. J Reprod Fertil Suppl 1975;135–7.
36. Patil PS, Humbarwadi RS, Patil AD, et al. Immature germ cells in semen – correlation with total sperm count and sperm motility. J Cytol 2013;30:185–9.
37. Goyal H. Histoquantitative effects of orchiectomy with and without testosterone enanthate treatment on the bovine epididymis. Am J Vet Res 1983;44:1085–90.
38. Coulter GH, Cook RB, Kastelic JP. Effects of dietary energy on scrotal surface temperature, seminal quality, and sperm production in young beef bulls. J Anim Sci 1997;75:1048–52.
39. Barth AD, Cates WF, Harland RJ. The effect of amount of body fat and loss of fat on breeding soundness classification of beef bulls. Can Vet J 1995;36:758–64.
40. Palmer CW. Management and breeding soundness of mature bulls. Vet Clin North Am Food Anim Pract 2016;32:479–95.
41. Koziol JH, Palmer CW. Pathophysiology, diagnosis, and management of testicular degeneration in the bull. Clin Therio 2023;15:9271.
42. Randel RD, Chase CC Jr, Wyse SJ. Effects of gossypol and cottonseed products on reproduction of mammals. J Anim Sci 1992;70:1628–38.
43. Chenoweth P, Chase C, Risco C, et al. Characterization of gossypol-induced sperm abnormalities in bulls. Theriogenology 2000;53:1193–203.
44. Chenoweth PJ, Risco CA, Larsen RE, et al. Effects of dietary gossypol on aspects of semen quality, sperm morphology and sperm production in young Brahman bulls. Theriogenology 1994;42:1–13.
45. Chenoweth PJ. Genetic sperm defects. Theriogenology 2005;64:457–68.

# Ancillary Methods for Semen Evaluation

Jennifer H. Koziol, DVM, MS*

## KEYWORDS

- Semen evaluation • Bulls • Ancillary • Sperm morphology

## KEY POINTS

- The cause of subfertility or poor fertility in naturally mated bulls should be differentiated from impotentia coeundi, generandi, or erigendi prior to ancillary semen evaluation.
- Bulls used for artificial insemination may undergo ancillary semen evaluation following low fertility rates as judged by poor conception or low pregnancy rates.
- Morphologically abnormal sperm have long been associated with bull subfertility and infertility. Some morphological defects such as improper sperm chromatin condensation are not visible using traditional light microscopy and require specialized staining.
- Ancillary semen evaluation is useful in cases where the reason for low or absence of fertility needs to be identified.

## INTRODUCTION

Morphologically abnormal sperm have long been associated with male infertility and assessment of these abnormalities is a fundamental component of analysis of semen quality.[1–4] Sperm morphology is an excellent predictor of the outcome of natural mating, artificial insemination, and *in vitro* fertilization[4–6] and there is a relationship between morphologically abnormal sperm and poor DNA quality.[3]

Traditional evaluation of sperm morphology either by brightfield or phase contrast allows for the identification of head, midpiece, and principal piece defects. Brightfield microscopy is suitable for the examination of morphology utilizing stained semen smears. Morphology evaluations must always be performed using the oil immersion (100X) objective lens; with eyepieces of 10 to 12.5X, the total magnification is 1000 to 1250X (hereafter referred to as 1000X). Morphology evaluation at lower magnification is not recommended as it results in failure to recognize many sperm abnormalities.

Utilization of phase contrast microscopy allows the examination of unstained, cover-slipped, preparations prepared by mixing semen with warmed 10% neutral buffered formalin on a microscope slide, as well as slides stained with Feulgen stain.[7]

---

Texas Tech School of Veterinary Medicine, 7671 Evans Drive, Amarillo, TX 79106, USA
* Corresponding author.
*E-mail address:* jkoziol@ttu.edu

Vet Clin Food Anim 40 (2024) 41–49
https://doi.org/10.1016/j.cvfa.2023.06.002
0749-0720/24/© 2023 Elsevier Inc. All rights reserved.

Evaluation of sperm morphology utilizing phase contrast at 1000X is preferred over the use of stained preparations by some practitioners, as defects such as nuclear vacuoles,[8] acrosomal defects, and abnormal DNA in the case of Feulgen stained slides are easier to identify. However, these defects can also readily be identified with high-quality brightfield microscopes. It also should be noted that phase-contrast slides should be allowed to settle for 15 minutes prior to observation to prevent sperm cells from laying in multiple planes and consequently creating the artifact of misshapen or narrow-based heads.[9,10]

Despite careful and thorough evaluation of sperm morphology by a veterinarian a producer may notice a bull experiencing unexpected subfertility or infertility. These bulls are often identified by excessive numbers of returns-to-estrus or excessive non-pregnant cows at the time of pregnancy examination, reduced calving rates, or may even be identified following parentage verification in multi-sire pastures. If the bull warrants further work up the veterinarian should work through a differential list of potential reasons for subfertility/infertility including impotentia coeundi, impotentia erigendi and impotentia generandi. Impotentia coeundi is defined as an inability or unwillingness to copulate. Impotentia generandi is characterized by normal libido and normal ability to copulate but subfertility or infertility. Impotentia erigendi is defined as the inability to achieve or maintain an erection of the penis.

Impotentia coeundi and erigendi can commonly be ruled out following a test mating. Once impotentia generandi is identified as the most likely cause for the subfertility/infertility and routine semen evaluation including motility and morphology assessment by bright-field or phase microscopy does not identify the problem and infectious diseases testing has occurred ancillary semen evaluation may be warranted to identify the issue(s). Owners may request ancillary semen tests to isolate and define the issue either for genetic or insurance purposes.

Similarly, in the artificial insemination industry bulls with poor fertility based on poor conception rates in inseminated cows may undergo further analysis to identify issues for similar reasons as mentioned above.[11]

The following ancillary methods for semen evaluation are divided into those that can be done in the clinic followed by those that likely will have to be sent to a supporting diagnostic or andrology lab due to the requirement for specialized equipment.

## FEULGEN STAINING

In the early stages of spermatogenesis, sperm DNA is associated with large basic histone nucleoproteins similar to other somatic cells. However, during the final stages of spermatogenesis, sperm chromatin structure is modified and as spermiogenesis proceeds, histones are initially replaced by transition proteins which are subsequently replaced by small protamines.[12] This substitution of protamine allows DNA chains to lie parallel to each other to facilitate the formation of a compact nucleus, resistant to denaturation. Incomplete condensation and partial retention of histones results in sperm malfunction.[13]

Abnormal DNA condensation cannot be detected by standard light microscopic examination of unstained semen preparations or in routinely stained preparations that do not specifically identify chromosomal material or DNA. When infertility or subfertility is observed in healthy animals with adequate semen quality, libido and mating ability, abnormal DNA condensation may explain fertilization failure.

A practical way to assess DNA condensation is Feulgen staining, which allows visual microscopic detection of abnormal DNA condensation.[4] In the Feulgen reaction, aldehyde groups in the deoxyribose component of DNA are unmasked by acid hydrolysis and then exposed to Schiff's reagent.[13] Normal sperm nuclei appear a homogenous purplish red with brightfield microscopy and intensely violet with phase microscopy at 1000X. In contrast, abnormal DNA condensation usually appears as coarse or fine clumping of nuclear material with a generalized reduced staining intensity of the nucleus. Affected nuclei often have an expanded appearance. In some cases, nuclei appear slightly mottled and pale. Nuclear vacuolation may be associated with abnormal sperm condensation. Concurrent control samples should always be used to confirm abnormal DNA staining with the Feulgen and other staining techniques.[13] The existence of clumped granular chromatin has also been detected with electron microscopy. Feulgen and SCSA methods have been compared and the 2 methods have good correlation with the proportion of affected sperm and with fertility.[14] Feulgen staining can be performed in the clinic and the supplies are readily available through companies that supply scientific chemicals and supplies. The method for Feulgen staining can be found later in discussion in **Box 1**.

## SPERMAC STAIN

Spermac stain (Minitube USA, Inc. Verona, WI) has been advocated as a specialized stain to evaluate the acrosome region of the sperm utilizing light microscopy as compared to the more time-consuming and costly methods of acrosome evaluation by fluorescent microscopy or flow cytometry. Acrosome integrity is important as the acrosome is essential for the penetration of sperm into the zona pellucida and resulting fertilization. Spermac stain consists of a fixative followed by 3 distinct stains. Following staining, slides can be evaluated at 1000X, and the acrosome region of the sperm can be easily assessed. In normal sperm the anterior region of the acrosome is stained green with a darker green halo forming an unbroken semicircle at the tip of the head. The posterior acrosome region of each sperm will have a red-pink coloration. If the red-pink color is not present the sperm cell was not adequately stained and should not be evaluated. Sperm with reacted or flawed acrosomes show peeling acrosome membranes, irregular thicknesses in the green halo along the tip of the head or partial green coloration. Those sperm with non-intact acrosomes will stain either white or red at the acrosomal region with no green color at the head. To date, no published studies have investigated a difference between Spermac versus traditional evaluation techniques regarding the ability to identify certain acrosome defects.

---

**Box 1**
**Feulgen staining protocol**

Materials Needed
- Gloves
- 5N HCL
- Dried semen smears
- Schiff's reagent

Protocol
1. Schiff's reagent can cause severe skin burns and is suspected of causing cancer consequently gloves should be worn.
2. Dip dried slides in 5N HCL for 45 minutes
3. Rinse slides in running tap water for 30 seconds following removal from 5N HCL.
4. Dip slides into Schiff's reagent for 45 minutes.
   a. Schiff's reagent should be changed every 2 weeks for best results.
5. Rinse slides in running tap water for 30 seconds following from Schiff's reagent.
6. Allow slides to air dry and then review slides with phase contrast microscopy.

## HYPO-OSMOTIC SWELLING TESTING

Hypo-osmotic swelling test (HOS test) also known as osmotic resistance tests (ORT) is a useful test for determining sperm quality and evaluating the membrane integrity of spermatozoa. Functional membrane integrity is a prerequisite for fertilizing ability of spermatozoa as it plays an integral role in sperm capacitation. Membrane integrity can be evaluated by the commonly used supravital stains such as eosin-nigrosin which stains all cells without an intact plasma membrane red. HOS testing has been described as being superior to supravital staining due as it tests the ability of the plasma membrane to be biochemically sound and to be able to functionally react appropriately to the testing whereas supravital stain only determines if the membrane is intact or not.[15]

HOS testing is a simple and economical test which aids in the evaluation of the structural and functional integrity of the sperm. This test works on basis that liquid diffuses across the cell membrane of the sperm cell under hypo-osmotic conditions in order to reach equilibrium on both sides of the cell membrane. Due to this influx of fluid into the cell reflex of the midpiece and coiling of the tail occurs in normal sperm. The swelling ability of the plasma membrane during the hypo-osmotic test is indicative of functional spermatozoa.

The standard method for testing raw semen consists of incubating 5-10 µL of semen in 1 mL of 150 mOsm kg$^{-1}$ solution for 40-60 minutes at a temperature of 35°C. If one is wishing to assess post-thaw extended semen the osmolality should be adjusted to 100 mOsm kg$^{-1}$; all other parameters remain the same. The solution is made from a mixture of fructose and trisodium citrate. Following the incubation period an aliquot of the semen in the solution is taken and placed on warm, clean microscope slide and cover slipped. The slide can then be evaluated at 400X either with brightfield or phase contrast microscopy. A heated stage is preferred. Cells are considered to have swollen or reacted if they have a reflex of the midpiece or tail or coiling of the tail indicating that the plasma membrane is functional. A minimum of 100 cells should be counted with the examiner counting the number of sperm cells that show signs of swelling or no reaction.[16]

## DIFFERENTIAL INTERFERENCE CONTRAST MICROSCOPY

Differential interface contrast microscopy (DIC) is considered the gold standard for evaluating sperm morphology by light microscopy and gives a three-dimensional appearance to viewed sperm. Nonetheless, due to the cost-prohibitive nature of this type of microscopy it usually is only found in well-equipped andrology labs.

DIC utilizes wet-mount slides with cells being evaluated in a unfixed or fixed status.[4,17] DIC slides are frequently prepared with buffered formol saline. Sperm cells appear bright with a dark background with no diffraction halo artifact which is often noted with the observation of sperm cells utilizing phase contrast. DIC provides the viewer with the clear visualization of the acrosome and sperm head in general. Minute defects of the head such as diadem defects as well as acrosome defects are best visualized with this light microscope system.

In an experiment comparing DIC to eosin-nigrosin stained sperm cells; the use of DIC was statistically determined to be better suited for identifying acrosome defects and diadem/vacuoles/pouch defects as shown by the statistically significant increase of abnormal sperm identified with those characteristics as compared to the evaluation of an eosin-nigrosin stained semen slide from the same bull.[18] It should be noted though that no difference was found in the percent of normal cells identified over-all by the evaluators using bright-field or DIC. Bright-field assessment of eosin-nigrosin prepared slides was equally effective in assessing the potential breeder status of a bull.[18] Evaluation of semen by DIC can be performed in referral cases where the expert evaluation of semen morphology is warranted.

## COMPUTER-ASSISTED SPERM ANALYSIS

Computer Assisted Sperm Analysis (CASA), a computer-based technique, has become increasingly more popular, especially in andrology labs and semen processing laboratories. CASA allows for the objective measurement of concentration, sperm motility, and kinematic motion including velocity, linearity, and lateral displacement of the head which defines the trajectory of the sperm. This machine allows for thousands of sperm within a sample to be evaluated and assessed. This technique uses continuous imaging of motile sperm to create video images at which point a software program assigns sperm into subgroups based on motion. While often thought to be entirely automated these machines are not ready-to-use and standardization of use is necessary.[19] Sample preparation, chamber type, and debris or extender within the semen sample are all factors that must be controlled when evaluating semen in such a manner.

Donnelly and colleagues[20] noted a significant difference in the observed motility parameters between sperm that achieved a high percentage of fertilization as compared to those failed to achieve a viable pregnancy. Furthermore, Budworth and colleagues[21,22] observed significant correlations between progressive motility and spermatozoon velocity when compared to competitive fertility indexes. Similar results were shown by Farrell and colleagues,[23] Januskauskas and colleagues[24] and Kathiravan and colleagues[25] Collectively, these articles point to the fact that the characterization of sperm motion especially progressive motility and velocity parameters can be useful in predicting potential fertility in bull semen. In the bull, motility and membrane integrity are often highly correlated with sperm morphology characteristics and consequently those bulls with better progressive motility and velocity likely have more normal sperm as compared to those bulls which do not.

## FLOW CYTOMETRY

Flow cytometry is a highly specialized piece of equipment that can be used for the evaluation of many sperm cells in a short period. It is composed of fluidics, optics, and an electronics system which measures physical optics and chemical fluorescence characteristics of stained sperm cells in fluid as they pass a laser source.[26] Based on the fluorescent emission the system generates high-throughput data.

Sperm cells can be labeled with a multitude of fluorescent markers that can be used to highlight certain structures within the sperm cell and allow for the characterization of normal or abnormal. Later in discussion we will discuss the types of analyses that can be performed by flow cytometry.

### Cell Viability Analysis

Cell viability analysis identifies viable and non-viable sperm which is associated with the plasma membrane. Multiple fluorescent probes can be used for this method with propidium iodide being one of the most commonly used. Propidium iodide can penetrate non-viable cells through the broken plasmalemma and will emit as red once excited by the laser. SYBR-14 is also often used in conjunction with propidium iodide. SYBR-14, a viability probe, emits green fluorescence from nuclei upon entering active cells. Consequently, when used together cells that are non-viable are stained red and viable cells are stained green.

### Acrosome Integrity

Flow cytometry can access sperm for intact acrosomes by labeling the acrosomes with lectin probes conjugated with fluorochrome fluorescent isothiocyanate (FITC). In damaged acrosome they will emit a green fluorescence while intact acrosomes yield no fluorescence. The acrosome and membrane integrity can be measure at the same time with the addition of propidium iodide.[27,28]

### Mitochondrial Activity

As an indicator of sperm physiology mitochondrial function can be assessed by flow cytometry. Mito Tracker or JC-1 dyes, both dyes that permeate the cell and accumulate in the mitochondria allow for the quantification of the mitochondrial membrane potential (MMP). JC-1 is more specific to MMP with fluorescence shifting from green to orange showing differences in the sperm mitochondrial function.[29]

### Sperm Chromatin Structure Assay

Sperm chromatin structure assays (SCSA) can be used to evaluate the character of chromatin in individual sperm and is considered the gold standard for measuring DNA damage.[30] Sperm chromatin structure assays involve acridine orange staining and assessment by flow cytometry to measure the susceptibility of sperm chromatin to acid-induced denaturation.[31] Double-stranded DNA will fluoresce green while single-stranded DNA emits a red fluorescence. The amount of DNA fragmentation noted in a sample has been shown to be correlated to fertility in the bull.[32-35]

## ELECTRON MICROSCOPY

Electron microscopy utilizes a beam of accelerated electrons to produce a specimen image. This technique provides higher magnification and resolution than light microscopy and allows for the visualization of the internal structures, ultrastructure, and morphological characteristics of sperm cells.[36] The 2 most common electron microscopes are transmission electron microscopy (TEM) and scanning electron microscope (SEM). With these advanced microscopes the electron beam is focused on the specimen. TEM creates a two-dimensional image while SEM creates a three-dimensional image. SEM is advantageous when investigating adverse effects of cryopreservation on sperm morphological changes[37] while TEM is applicable to deep investigation of structure and function of sperm as the entire structure of the sperm cell can be visualized and is the best method for the study of teratozoospermia.[38]

TEM can be extremely useful for identifying minuscule acrosome defects, issues with the chromatin, and centrosome defects. These issues are difficult if not impossible to identify by light microscopy with the exception of chromatin structure which was discussed above. Midpiece and tail defects including sperm mitochondrial anomalies, axoneme defects including microtubule malformations, and periaxonemal structure can also be evaluated by TEM. TEM is considered the gold standard method for the identification of midpiece and tail defects.[38]

## CLINICS CARE POINTS

- A thorough history and physical exam including a test mating should be completed on natural service bulls before ancillary semen testing is initiated.
- Simple tests such as Feulgen staining can occur in clinic and rarely necessitate the need to send to an outside laboratory.

• Discussion with owners regarding future use of the bull and necessity of the test to be performed will determine if the cost of diagnostic tests are warranted for an individual.

## DISCLOSURE

The author declares no conflicts of interest or sources of funding.

## REFERENCES

1. Kubo-Irie M, Matsumiya K, Iwamoto T, et al. Morphological abnormalities in the spermatozoa of fertile and infertile men. Mol Reprod Dev 2005;70:70–81.
2. Ostermeier GC, Sargeant GA, Yandell BS, et al. Relationship of bull fertility to sperm nuclear shape. J Androl 2001;22:595–603.
3. Enciso M, Cisale H, Johnston SD, et al. Major morphological sperm abnormalities in the bull are related to sperm DNA damage. Theriogenology 2011;76:23–32.
4. Barth AD, Oko RJ. Abnomal morphology of bovine spermatozoa. Malden: Blackwell Publishing Inc; 1989.
5. Wiltbank J, Parish N. Pregnancy rate in cows and heifers bred to bulls selected for semen quality. Theriogenology 1986;25:779–83.
6. Saacke R, Dalton J, Nadir S, et al. Relationship of seminal traits and insemination time to fertilization rate and embryo quality. Anim Reprod Sci 2000;60:663–77.
7. Sekoni V, Gustafsson B, Mather E. Influence of wet fixation, staining techniques, and storage time on bull sperm morphology. Nord Vet Med 1980;33:161–6.
8. Menon AG, Thundathil JC, Wilde R, et al. Validating the assessment of bull sperm morphology by veterinary practitioners. Can Vet J 2011;52:407–8.
9. Barth AD, Bowman PA, Bo GA, et al. Effect of narrow sperm head shape on fertility in cattle. Can Vet J 1992;33:31–9.
10. Thundathil J, Palasz AT, Mapletoft RJ, et al. An investigation of the fertilizing characteristics of pyriform-shaped bovine spermatozoa. Anim Reprod Sci 1999;57:35–50.
11. Fair S, Lonergan P. Review: Understanding the causes of variation in reproductive wastage among bulls. Animal 2018;12(Suppl 1):s53–62.
12. Ward WS, Coffey DS. DNA packaging and organization in mammalian spermatozoa: comparison with somatic cells. Biol Reprod 1991;44:569–74.
13. Barth AD. Bull breeding soundness. 3rd ed. Saskatoon: Western Canadian Association of Bovine Practitioners; 2013.
14. Dobrinski I, Hughes HP, Barth AD. Flow cytometric and microscopic evaluation and effect on fertility of abnormal chromatin condensation in bovine sperm nuclei. J Reprod Fertil 1994;101:531–8.
15. Zubair M, Ahmad M, Jamil H. Review on the screening of semen by hypo-osmotic swelling test. Andrologia 2015;47:744–50.
16. Revell SG, Mrode RA. An osmotic resistance test for bovine semen. Anim Reprod Sci 1994;36:77–86.
17. Saacke RG, Marshall CE. Observations on the acrosomal cap of fixed and unfixed bovine spermatozoa. J Reprod Fertil 1968;16:511–4.
18. Freneau GE, Chenoweth PJ, Ellis R, et al. Sperm morphology of beef bulls evaluated by two different methods. Anim Reprod Sci 2010;118:176–81.
19. Contri A, Valorz C, Faustini M, et al. Effect of semen preparation on casa motility results in cryopreserved bull spermatozoa. Theriogenology 2010;74:424–35.

20. Donnelly ET, Lewis SE, McNally JA, et al. In vitro fertilization and pregnancy rates: the influence of sperm motility and morphology on IVF outcome. Fertil Steril 1998; 70:305–14.

21. Budworth PR, Amann RP, Hammerstedt RH. A Microcomputer-photographic method for evaluation of motility and velocity of bull sperm. J Dairy Sci 1987; 70:1927–36.

22. Budworth PR, Amann RP, Chapman PL. Relationships between computerized Measurements of motion of frozen-thawed bull spermatozoa and fertility. J Androl 1988;9:41–54.

23. Farrell PB, Presicce GA, Brockett CC, et al. Quantification of bull sperm characteristics measured by computer-assisted sperm analysis (CASA) and the relationship to fertility. Theriogenology 1998;49:871–9.

24. Januskauskas A, Johannisson A, Söderquist L, et al. Assessment of sperm characteristics post-thaw and response to calcium ionophore in relation to fertility in Swedish dairy AI bulls. Theriogenology 2000;53:859–75.

25. Kathiravan P, Kalatharan J, Edwin MJ, et al. Computer automated motion analysis of crossbred bull spermatozoa and its relationship with in vitro fertility in zona-free hamster oocytes. Anim Reprod Sci 2008;104:9–17.

26. Givan AL. Flow cytometry: an introduction. Methods Mol Biol 2011;699:1–29.

27. Thomas CA, Garner DL, DeJarnette J, et al. Fluorometric sssessments of acrosomal integrity and viability in cryopreserved bovine spermatozoa. Biol Reprod 1997;56:991–8.

28. Graham JK, Kunze E, Hammerstedt RH. Analysis of sperm cell viability, acrosomal integrity, and mitochondrial function using flow cytometry. Biol Reprod 1990;43(1):55–64.

29. Garner DL, Thomas CA, Joerg HW, et al. Fluorometric assessments of mitochondrial function and viability in cryopreserved bovine spermatozoa. Biol Reprod 1997;57:1401–6.

30. Agarwal A and Said TM. Sperm chromatin assessment. Textbook of assisted reproductive techniques, In: Gardner DK, Weissman A, Howles C, Showham Z. Laboratory perspectives, vol. 1, 4th edition, 2012, CRC Press; Boca Raton, FL, 75–95.

31. Evenson DP. The Sperm chromatin structure assay (SCSA) and other sperm DNA fragmentation tests for evaluation of sperm nuclear DNA integrity as related to fertility. Anim Reprod Sci 2016;169:56–75.

32. Ballachey BE, Hohenboken WD, Evenson DP. Heterogeneity of sperm nuclear chromatin structure and its relationship to bull fertility. Biol Reprod 1987;36:915–25.

33. Ballachey BE, Evenson DP, Saacke RG. The sperm chromatin structure assay relationship with alternate tests of semen quality and heterospermic performance of bulls. J Androl 1988;9:109–15.

34. Sailer BL, Jost LK, Evenson DP. Mammalian sperm DNA susceptibility to in situ denaturation associated with the presence of DNA strand breaks as measured by the terminal deoxynucleotidyl transferase assay. J Andol 1995;16:80–7.

35. Waterhouse K, Haugan T, Kommisrud E, et al. Sperm DNA damage is related to field fertility of semen from young Norwegian Red bulls. Reprod Fertil Dev 2006; 18:781–8.

36. Sathananthan AH. Ultrastructure of human gametes, fertilization and embryos in assisted reproduction: a personal survey. Micron 2013;44:1–20.

37. Ozkavukcu S, Erdemli E, Isik A, et al. Effects of cryopreservation on sperm parameters and ultrastructural morphology of human spermatozoa. J Assist Reprod Genet 2008;25(8):403–11.
38. Moretti E, Sutera G, Collodel G. The importance of transmission electron microscopy analysis of spermatozoa: Diagnostic applications and basic research. Syst Biol Reprod Med 2016;62:171–83.

# Medical and Surgical Management of Conditions of the Penis and Prepuce

Chance L. Armstrong, DVM, MS*, Aubrey N. Baird, DVM, MS[1]

## KEYWORDS

- Urogenital surgery • Bulls • Prepuce • Laceration • Penis • Hematoma

## KEY POINTS

- Preputial and penile injuries in breeding bulls resulting in temporary loss of reproductive performance or culling are major sources of financial loss to the cow-calf operator.
- Conditions of the penis and prepuce that limit or prevent coitus emphasize the value of visualization and careful examination during the breeding soundness examination.
- Regional anesthesia combined with heavy sedation can provide a means for surgical procedures on marginally valued bulls.

## INTRODUCTION

The inability of a bull to reproduce due to its inability to impregnant fertile cows is called *impotentia generandi*. The resulting infertility may be due to the inability to achieve erection, *impotentia erigendi*, complete coitus, *impotentia coeundi*, or produce an adequate volume of morphologically normal, progressively motile spermatozoa. Reproductive failure due to bulls that fail to achieve coitus despite meeting the minimum standards of the Society for Theriogenology for the Bull Breeding Soundness Exam (BBSE) is a source of major financial loss for the beef and dairy industries. Therapies that target the urogenital tract of the bull can restore reproductive capabilities and preserve the significant investment incurred by producers annually. Veterinarians can provide consultation regarding management and selection criteria to help mitigate risk associated with some conditions of the penis and prepuce.

## EXAMINATION OF THE PENIS AND PREPUCE

Investigation of a bull that is unable to breed begins with a thorough history and physical examination including complete evaluation of the reproductive organs. Distance

Auburn University College of Veterinary Medicine, 1500 Wire Road, Auburn, AL 36849, USA
[1] Co author.
* Corresponding author.
*E-mail address:* armstcl@auburn.edu

Vet Clin Food Anim 40 (2024) 51–67
https://doi.org/10.1016/j.cvfa.2023.09.002
0749-0720/24/© 2023 Elsevier Inc. All rights reserved.

examination of the penis and prepuce should be followed by manual examination of the bull safely restrained in a chute. Conformation of the sheath is important. The distal end of the sheath should be no longer than a line drawn from the hock to the carpus (**Fig. 1** Line A). The distal end of the sheath, the preputial orifice, should not be excessively large, and the sheath angle should roughly approximate a line drawn parallel along the ventral aspect of the sheath, that intersects the distal limb or hoof (see **Fig. 1** Line B). Adequate restraint within a chute is critical for further evaluation of the bull. With the bull in a chute moderate side squeeze should be applied and a sturdy bar placed behind him to limit kicking during examination. In a healthy bull, preputial hairs should be free of calculi, exudate, or hemorrhage. The penis and prepuce should be contained within the sheath. Naturally polled bulls may have a slight prolapse of the prepuce when relaxed. The entire length of the penis should be palpated through the sheath for swelling or fibrous tissue. Preputial abscessation and penile hematomas can cause palpable focal swelling. Location and symmetry of swelling can be used to distinguish the most likely pathology. Preputial abscesses are usually well circumscribed swellings along the midportion (half-way between the preputial orifice and the scrotum) of the sheath. Penile hematomas produce symmetrical swelling on the dorsum of the penis at the distal bend of the sigmoid flexure (just cranial to the scrotum). Retropreputial abscesses share a similar location to penile hematomas but differ in asymmetrical swelling. Preputial lacerations can result in generalized swelling spanning the entire length of the sheath. This swelling is the result of cellulitis associated with the laceration or secondary to urine contamination of the peripenile elastic tissue.

Visual examination of the penis is critical. The penis can be manually extended with the aid of an assistant. Once extended, the free portion of the penis should be grasp with a dry surgical sponge and gently separated from the surrounding prepuce. The skin of the penis should be moist and pink devoid of any swelling, vesicles, pustules, papillomas, lacerations, or scar tissue.

## ABNORMALITIES OF THE PENIS AND PREPUCE
### Juvenile Anomalies of the Penis and Prepuce

#### Persistent frenulum
Persistent frenulum consists of a congenital band-like attachment of the prepuce from the tip of the free portion of the penis along the median raphe to the base of the free portion of the preputial epithelium. The bands may be thick and broad or

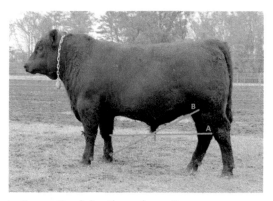

**Fig. 1.** Bull demonstrating optimal sheath conformation.

thin containing one or more blood vessels. Usually identified in virgin bulls during the initial breeding soundness examination. The frenulum should not be confused with incomplete separation of the penis and preputial epithelium. The frenulum impairs full extension of the penis and prepuce. A sharp ventral deviation of the erect penis is often noted. Impotence induced by this condition in *Bos taurus* bulls may not affect *Bos indicus* bulls due to the excessive length of prepuce.[1] Nonetheless, in some cases, this condition may be confused with phimosis. This is particularly true in bulls with excessively redundant preputial skin, if the ventral bending of the prepuce prevents extension of the glans beyond the preputial orifice.[2] Evidence of heritability recommends culling affected bulls from purebred herds or restricting their use as a terminal sire only.[3] Otherwise, the frenulum is easily ligated at each end and excised with the bull restrained in a chute or on a tilt-table (**Fig. 2**).[4] The authors suggest that bulls return for reevaluation 30 days postoperatively to confirm that full extension can be achieved.

### Incomplete separation of the penis and prepuce

The surface epithelium of the free portion of the penis is firmly attached to the preputial epithelium of the prepuce at birth limiting preputial extension. The interdigitating attachment gradually begins to separate at 1 month of age and proceeds caudally until complete separation between 8 and 11 months of age to facilitate complete penile extension at puberty.[5,6] Sporadically, this separation occurs prematurely in young bulls as a result of hematoma formation from hemorrhage between surface epithelial layers after attempts to mount and extend the penis. Treatment is strictly symptomatic. Surgical intervention is not indicated. In rare cases, if bacteria should gain entry to the damaged tissues, an abscess may result in adhesions or phimosis.[2] Normal separation is sometimes delayed in yearling bulls resulting in an inability to fully extend the penis at the time of a breeding soundness examination or during an observed mating. If given time to fully mature, the attachment will regress. However, separation especially in cases of partial separation following electroejaculation, may be aided with gentle separation of the interdigitating layers. Hemorrhage is often observed when forced separation of the penis and prepuce occurs during the BBSE (**Fig. 3**) Bulls should be placed in the deferred category if there is assistance in the separation of the interdigital layers and rechecked in 2 to 4 weeks to ensure that no adhesions were formed from the forced separation.

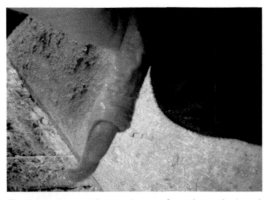

**Fig. 2.** Yearling bull presenting with persistent frenulum during breeding soundness examination.

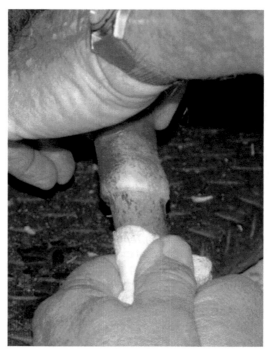

**Fig. 3.** Manual separation of partial attachment of the penis and prepuce in a young bull.

### Hair rings

Bulls, especially young bulls, may display a matted ring of hair surrounding the free portion of the penis. The hair comes from body coat hair of other bulls that have been mounted by the aggressor or from their own preputial orifice during masturbation. The ring should be removed to avoid a deep annular laceration leading to the creation of a urethral fistula, cavernosal fistula, or eventually penile amputation (**Fig. 4**).

### Penile fibropapilloma

Viral papillomas or penile warts are found frequently on the penis and occasionally the prepuce of young bulls housed in groups. Abrasions allow entry of bovine papilloma

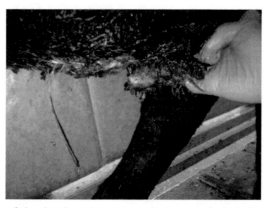

**Fig. 4.** Amputation of the distal penis as a sequela to a penile hair ring.

virus. Warts grow rapidly and may surround the tip of the penis causing phimosis or paraphimosis in some cases.[7] The growths may occur as a single, pedunculated growth near the glans penis, or as multiple or sessile growths.[8] Surgical removal is indicated with the preservation of the glans penis and urethra being of utmost importance. The bull is restrained either in a chute or on a tilt table. The penis is manually extended, and a towel clamp is placed under the apical ligament or a gauze tourniquet around the free portion of the penis to aid in penile extension. The penis is thoroughly scrubbed and 2 to -4 mL of 2% lidocaine is infiltrated subcutaneously across the dorsum of the penis proximal to the lesion. Surgical preparation is repeated and the urethra is carefully identified to avoid incising during removal of the growth. An 8 to 10-French, polypropylene catheter inserted into the urethra may assist the surgeon in avoiding the structure (**Fig. 5**). Large growths may need to be debulked to identify the base of the growth.[8] Once the base has been identified, careful dissection of the skin of the penis from the growth is required, making sure to remove all fibrous tissue. Ligation of any small vessels and closure of the skin can be performed with chromic gut or poliglecaprone 25. The towel clamp is removed, and the penis is allowed to retract into the preputial cavity. The author does not regularly recommend topical or systemic antimicrobials postoperatively. Use of commercial or autogenous wart vaccine has been suggested to reduce reoccurrence of lesions and as a preventative in bulls entering development lots.[9] Bulls treated for penile fibropapillomas should be reexamined in 4 weeks for healing and potential regrowth. The authors have observed the administration of immunostimulants (mycobacterium cell wall fraction) at surgery may help prevent recurrence of penile warts.

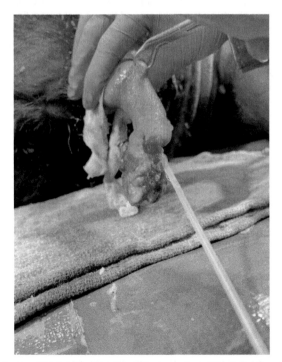

**Fig. 5.** Penile wart associated with the glans penis and positioning of an 8-French polypropylene catheter in the urethra for surgeon reference. Towel clamp placement under the dorsal apical ligament to hold the penis in extension.

### Anatomic and Developmental Anomalies

#### Penile deviations
Deviation of the normal shape of the erect penis inhibits the ability to copulate. Three types of penile deviations in decreasing order of occurrence are spiral or corkscrew, ventral or rainbow, and S-shaped.[10] Affected bulls usually have one or more success-ful breeding seasons followed by one or more unsuccessful breeding seasons. Most affected bulls are 2.5 to 5 years of age.[11] Histories rarely indicate previous traumatic penile injury.

Originating from the tunica albuginea proximal to the free portion of the penis, the dorsal apical ligament runs along the dorsum of the free portion of the penis beneath the penile skin and rejoins the tunica albuginea near the distal end of the corpus cav-ernosum penis (CCP). The ligaments insert on the distal penis centrally with a broad set of fibers. The fibers of the dorsal apical ligament are heavier and less pliable on the left side than on the right.[6,12] The ligament gives support to the erect penis and maintains normal penile alignment for intromission. Following intromission and achievement of peak erectile pressure, the distal penis will sometimes assume a cork-screw shape and spiral within the vagina at the time of the ejaculatory lunge. These observations were confirmed using a transparent artificial vagina to collect semen. Most bulls exhibited spiraling within the artificial vagina to some extent but not at every service.[13]

Usually, abnormal spiraling is seen after penile protrusion; however, in some bulls, spiraling may occur within the preputial cavity.[14] For spiraling to occur, the thick fibers of the dorsal apical ligament must slip off the dorsum of the penis down on the left side of the ventrally bending glans penis; the ligament then pulls the tip of the penis back into the spiral. The thin fibers on the right side of the dorsal apical ligament stretch over the bend in the penis. It should be noted that spiraling during electroejaculation is iat-rogenic and has not been correlated with the tendency to spiral during natural service.

#### Spiral deviations of the penis
Pathologic spiral deviations of the penis occur when the dorsal apical ligament slips laterally to the left before intromission. Elements leading to the hasty occurrence of this otherwise normal phenomenon are poorly understood.[6,12,15] Malfunction of the dorsal apical ligament due to a shortening of the ligament or lengthening of the penis as the bull ages was once commonly thought to be the case but the theory remains unproven. More recently, the hypothesis that peak erectile pressures are reached prematurely before intromission has occurred resulting in premature spiraling of the glans penis.[11] Regardless of the cause, bulls with premature spiral deviation of the penis are unable to complete the copulatory act. Diagnosis of spiral deviation should only be made after observation during a test mating (**Fig. 6**). This condition is deceptive because the deviation may not consistently occur, especially in the early stages.

There is no medical treatment available to correct spiral deviation of the penis. Sur-gical correction of spiral deviation entails using a fascia lata graft or synthetic mesh that is secured on the dorsal surface of the tunica albuginea to strengthen the dorsal apical ligament attachment preventing premature spiral deviation of the penis.[8,16–18]

#### Ventral deviation of the penis
Ventral deviation of the penis is less common than spiral deviation. The exact cause is unknown; however, there is speculation that deviation results from a combination of altered architecture of the penile tunica albuginea or apical ligament and altered blood flow through the ventral portion of CCP. Both suspected causes are likely the result of

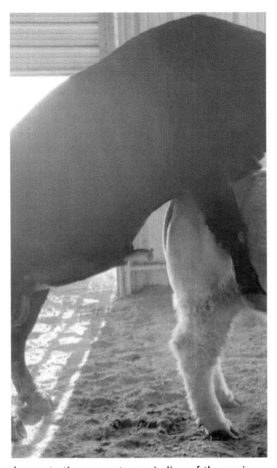

**Fig. 6.** Test mating demonstrating premature spiraling of the penis.

chronic traumatic injury.[8] The penis assumes a long gradual ventral curvature as erection progresses frequently originating proximal to the junction of the sheath and prepuce and becomes more evident as erection increases. This condition is often referred to as a "rainbow" due to the arc formed by the erect penis. Ventral deviation can be highly suspected during electroejaculation but a test breeding is recommended. Surgical correction of ventral deviation of the penis is less likely to be successful than the correction of the spiral deviation. Surgical intervention should only be attempted in cases of a ventral deviation if the deviation does not originate proximal to the free portion of the penis and is limited to the free portion of the penis.[8,19]

### S-shaped deviation of the penis
The S-shaped curvature of the penis is the least common of the deviations caused by inadequate apical ligament function. This condition usually occurs in bulls 4 years of age or older and is thought to be caused by inadequate apical ligament length or excessive penile length with a normal apical ligament. The condition may develop following trauma to the apical ligament with subsequent contracture and shortening of the ligament. Some bulls with this condition may be able to breed successfully.[11] No therapy is recommended for this condition. A bull with high genetic value could

have semen collected for artificial insemination purposes if the deviation prevents intromission.

## Acquired Conditions of the Penis and Prepuce

### Penile hematoma

The term hematoma of the penis is used to indicate rupture of the penile tunica albuginea. This condition is also referred to as broken or fractured penis. The physiology of erection and breeding behavior of the bull explains why and how rupture of the penis occurs. At the time of erection, venous outflow to the CCP is obstructed and contraction of the ischiocavernosus muscles increases pressure within the penis to approximately 14,199 mm Hg.[20,21] The bull mounts, makes 1 to 2 searching motions with the penis to locate the vulva, and achieves intromission and ejaculation with one forceful lunge. If the bull misses the vulva and hits the perineal area of the female or the female collapses during the mounting, severe angulation of the penile shaft may occur decreasing the volume of the CCP and drastically increasing the intrapenile pressure to greater than 70,000 mm Hg resulting in rupture of the tunica albuginea.[22] The most common site for rupture is on the dorsal surface of the distal sigmoid flexure just above the point of insertion of the paired retractor muscles, although in rare instances, it may occur at other locations.[23,24] The injury typically occurs early in the breeding season when a larger number of cows may be cycling, and the bull displays an excellent libido with the novelty of the cows. Alternatively, the injury may happen late in the breeding season when the bull can experience fatigue and becomes careless during coitus.

The erect penis contains less than 250 mL of blood at the time of rupture of the tunica albuginea. This blood under pressure forcefully enters the peripenile elastic tissue, creating a symmetric swelling in the sheath immediately cranial to the base of the scrotum. The hematoma may grow from comparatively small to quite large if repeated sexual stimulation results in additional attempts at erection and continued leakage of blood through the rent in the tunica albuginea.

Hematoma of the penis is diagnosed based on physical examination findings and must be differentiated from retropreputial abscess as previously described. Mild-to-moderate prolapse of the prepuce, which may have a distinct bluish tent secondary to the subcutaneous blood, is often the first sign of injury. Palpation of the distal bend of the sigmoid flexure of the penis will confirm rupture of the tunica albuginea. The penis will not extend because of swelling within the elastic tissues. Manual extension of the penis should not be atempted. Such efforts may tear the already injured elastic tissues. Use of electroejaculation is also contraindicated in cases of penile hematoma. Forced erection results in blood exiting the rent in the corpus cavernosum which can lead to enlargement of the hematoma.

Rupture of the tunica albuginea, while not life threatening may result in the loss of reproductive function. Potential complication following penile hematoma include abscess formation at the site of the hematoma, adhesions between the penis and peripenile tissues, development of vascular shunts between the CCP and surrounding vasculature, injury to the prolapsed tissues, and destruction of the dorsal nerves of the penis.[2] Approximately 50% of bulls with rupture of the tunica albuginea of the penis will resume breeding without surgical repair of the injured penis.[8] Conservative therapy consisting of forced sexual rest for at least 60 days combined with medical management is warranted when diagnosis is delayed, or the economic value of the bull does not justify the expense of surgery. Prophylactic systemic antibiotic therapy may reduce the risk of abscessation of the hematoma. Hydrotherapy of the sheath stimulates circulation to the damaged tissue, aids in resorption of the blood clot, and reduces the edema of the elastic tissues. If present, the prolapsed prepuce may be protected with an emollient ointment and support bandages as needed. The bull should undergo a complete breeding soundness examination before return to service.

More aggressive surgical correction results in approximately 80% of bulls returning to breeding soundness if surgery is performed promptly after the injury and if the prepuce is not seriously damaged. Surgery is recommended between 3 and 7 days following injury. Owners should be counseled that even following successful management and resolution, recurrence of injury may occur during subsequent breeding attempts.

### Eversion of the prepuce

Eversion of the prepuce is found to some degree in all bulls carrying the polled gene and/or B indicus breeds but not in horned bulls. Polled bulls lack the paired retractor prepuce muscles.[25,26] The lack of paired retractor prepuce muscles combined with the pendulousness of the sheath, the length of the internal lamina of the prepuce, and the size of the sheath opening are also factors that contribute to eversion of the prepuce or preputial prolapse (**Fig. 7**).[27] Bulls with a high degree of eversion are more subject to preputial trauma (eg, frostbite and lacerations).[27]

### Preputial lacerations

Bulls with pendulous sheath and excessive preputial skin may traumatize the preputial tissues independent of the breeding act. Most commonly penile lacerations in all breeds of bulls occur at the time of the ejaculatory lunge. As the free portion of the penis enters the vagina, preputial skin slides caudally up the shaft of the penis and folds of redundant skin gather at the preputial orifice forming a collar. Bunching of preputial skin usually occurs without incident but when the preputial tissue becomes

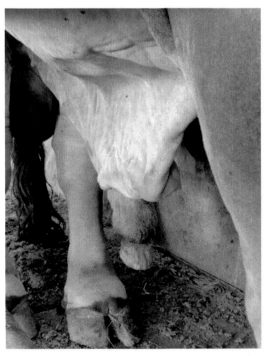

**Fig. 7.** Eversion of the prepuce that may develop trauma to exposed elastic tissue.

trapped between the bull's abdomen and the bony pelvis of the cow it may become traumatized by the compressive forces. In mild cases, the preputial epithelium remains intact and accumulation of edema in the damaged tissues results in an uncomplicated preputial prolapse. More serious injury occurs when compression of the entrapped prepuce causes bursting of the epithelium with subsequent exposure and damage of the underlying elastic tissues.[28] Lacerations of the prepuce with subsequent preputial prolapse is more common in B indicus breeds and their crosses than bulls of B taurus breeds. B indicus bulls with excessively pendulous sheaths, excess length of prepuce, and/or large preputial orifices are far more likely to sustain an injury than bulls lacking excessive skin in these areas. Preputial injuries in bulls of B taurus breeding often do not result in prolapse of the prepuce.[8]

Laceration or rupture of the epithelium of the prepuce predictably occurs longitudinal to the long axis of the ventral aspect of the prepuce but assumes a transverse orientation as the bull retracts the penis into the preputial cavity. The transverse orientation of the laceration effectively shortens the length of the traumatized tissue.[8] B taurus breeds usually retract the damaged prepuce back into the preputial cavity allowing the injury to go unnoticed until cellulitis, abscessation, or stenosis occurs. Retropreputial abscessation is a common sequala in this population of bulls. Phlegmon may extend from the external preputial orifice or maybe limited to a small, well-defined area along that sheath (**Fig. 8**). In contrast, edema may accumulate in the traumatized tissue causing prolapse of the prepuce most commonly in B indicus type bulls. The dependent edema increases the size and weight of the prolapsed tissue leading to prolapse of additional length of prepuce worsening the condition (**Fig. 9**).[2] This condition is most severe in naturally polled bulls, regardless of breed due to the lack of retractor prepuce muscles.[25,26] These muscles naturally serve to elevate the prepuce, and this elevation can minimize edema formation in damaged tissues.

Wolfe and Carson have constructed a 4-point classification scale that incorporates severity of the preputial injury to estimate prognosis for return to function and guide treatment decisions (**Table 1**). Desrochers and workers examined data from 51 bulls and discovered prognosis for return to breeding soundness following surgical intervention was 88% versus 36% if the penis could be extended during the initial evaluation of a preputial injury.[29] This prognostic data may be important to communicate to clients when considering surgery on a bull of marginal value relative to surgical costs.

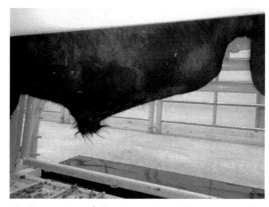

**Fig. 8.** Retropreputial abscessation following preputial trauma and retraction within the sheath.

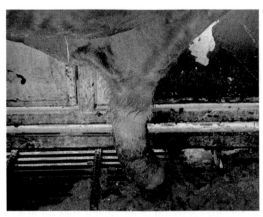

**Fig. 9.** Grade 3 preputial prolapse and effective shortening of the ventral aspect of the prepuce following a breeding injury.

Medical management of preputial laceration and subsequent prolapse is aimed at control of sepsis, reduction of edema, and eventual return of the damaged tissues to the preputial cavity. Therapy begins with thorough cleaning and soaking of the wound with dilute antiseptic combined with gentle debridement of devitalized, necrotic tissue (**Fig. 10**). This is followed by application of lanolin-based emollients and topical antibiotics to prevent further desiccation and infection within tissues and should be combined with bandaging. Bandaging of the exposed prepuce must be done carefully making sure the bandage does not strangulate the tissue but applies sufficient compression to reduce edema. The bandage is applied following cleansing, debridement, and application of the emollient ointment. A latex tube is inserted into the preputial orifice to allow urine egress from the prepuce. Once the tube is correctly placed, an orthopedic stocking is placed over the exposed tissue followed by application of a snug elastic tape bandage beginning at the distal end of the prolapsed tissue and working up overlapping the tape as it advances up the prolapsed tissue, preputial orifice to the sheath where it can be adhered to haired skin (**Fig. 11**). In cases with excessive edema,

| Table 1 | | |
|---|---|---|
| **Wolfe and Carson classification scheme for preputial lacerations[8]** | | |
| **Category** | **Description** | **Treatment and Prognosis** |
| I | Simple preputial prolapse with slight-to-moderate edema without laceration, necrosis, or fibrosis | Respond well to conservative or surgical treatment with good prognosis |
| II | Prolapsed prepuce has moderate-to-severe edema, may have superficial lacerations or slight necrosis but no evidence of fibrosis | Surgery is recommended with a good to guarded prognosis |
| III | Severe edema of the prolapsed prepuce with deep lacerations, moderate necrosis, and slight fibrosis | Surgery is indicated and prognosis is guarded |
| IV | Prolapsed prepuce has been exposed for quite some time and has severe edema, deep lacerations, deep necrosis, fibrosis, and often abscess | Surgery and salvage by slaughter are the only options. Surgery carries a guarded to poor prognosis |

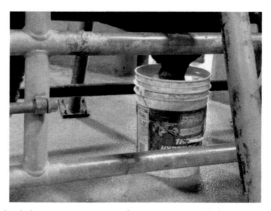

**Fig. 10.** Initial medical therapy consisting of an osmotic soak for at least 20 minutes.

a sling made of net or burlap material can be placed to allow the prepuce to be held close to the abdomen to encourage lymphatic flow and reduction of edema (**Fig. 12**). Frequent bandage changes are necessary. Prior to rebandaging, 15 to 20 minutes of hydrotherapy should be performed to help reduce edema and facilitate removal of devitalized tissue. Some bulls may return to service without surgery but recurrent injury is common.[8] Surgical resection and anastomosis (reefing or circumcision) of the preputial scar can improve outcome and is indicated when the bull's value exceeds the expense of this therapy. In the authors' opinion, this approach has provided the most positive outcomes compared with other methods that have been described. The surgery can be performed by restraint on a hydraulic tilt table with the application of general anesthesia or heavy sedation combined regional analgesia via internal pudendal nerve block (described in later discussion). The prepuce and penis are aseptically prepped with povidone scrub and saline. It is advised to prep the ventrum of the bull and place an impervious drape on the table to ensure proper sterility during the procedure. The defined scar is removed by making a circumferential incision proximal and distal to the scar and connecting with a longitudinal incision. The recommended preputial length is 1.5 times the length of the free portion of the penis after the scar is removed to ensure the bull can make full extension.[30] Damaged elastic tissueshould be removed using both sharp and blunt dissection.[30] The surgeon should strive to leave as much healthy

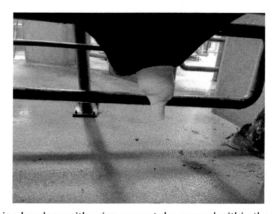

**Fig. 11.** Compression bandage with urine egress tube secured within the lumen of prepuce.

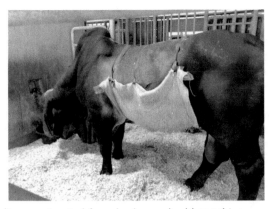

**Fig. 12.** Preputial sling constructed from burlap and rubber tubing.

elastic tissue as possible. Electrocautery is used for hemostasis along with ligation with 2-0 to #0 absorbable suture. Hemostasis and tissue handling are critical to achieve positive outcomes with this procedure. The author recommends lavage with saline infused with povidone solution before closure. The subcutaneous tissue is closed with #0 absorbable suture in quadrants to avoid a purse string effect and an increased risk of stricture of the lumen causing phimosis.[30] The skin can be closed in a similar manner or staples may be used (**Fig. 13**). Armstrong and Koziol, Unpublished data, 2016) is supportive of fewer surgical complications when staples are used to close the skin. A

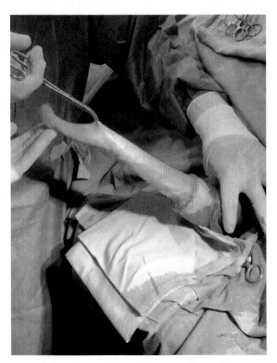

**Fig. 13.** Primary closure of the preputial epithelium with staples.

2.5-cm Penrose drain is sutured over the end of the glans penis to provide urine egress away from the incision. It is important to avoid the urethra on the ventral aspect of the penis when securing the drain. The penis and prepuce should be replaced back into the sheath and a rigid tube placed in the lumen with the aid of a lanolin-based emollient dressing on the proximal aspect. Large animal endotracheal tubes that are cut at different lengths provide enough support but are flexible enough to prevent stricture of the lumen for 3 to 5 days.[8] This tube can be secured by heavy elastic tape that is secured proximal to the hairline (see **Fig. 11**). Antibiotics and anti-inflammatory agents are administered for a period of 5 to 7 days postoperatively. The staples can be removed after 14 days. The surgery is always preceded by preoperative wound management as described above. The bull should have a BBSE completed after 60 days of strict sexual rest.

### Pudendal nerve block

An internal pudendal nerve block can provide analgesia for surgery of the penis or prepuce. To perform the block, begin by clipping and surgically preparing the skin at the ischiorectal fossa bilaterally. A caudal epidural is administered at a dose of 0.5 mL of 2% lidocaine hydrochloride per 100 pounds of body weight to desensitize the area. With the operator's left hand in the rectum, insert a 14-gauge, 1.25-cm needle is inserted through the desensitized skin at the ischiorectal fossa to serve as a cannula. An 18-gauge, 10 to 15 cm spinal needle is then directed through the cannula to the pudendal nerve (see **Fig. 14**). The operator's left hand is placed in the rectum to the level of the wrist and the fingers are directed laterally and ventrally to identify the right lesser sacrosciatic foramen.[31] The lesser sciatic foramen is first identified, and the internal pudendal nerve can be readily identified lying on the ligament immediately cranial and dorsal to the foramen and approximately one finger's width dorsal to the pudendal artery. This structure can be readily palpated a finger's width ventral to the nerve.[31] Once the pudendal nerve is located, 20 mL of local anesthetic is deposited around the nerve. The needle is partially withdrawn and relocated 2 to 3 cm more caudodorsally where an additional 10 mL of local anesthetic is deposited at the cranial aspect of the foramen to block the muscular branches and the middle hemorrhoidal nerves. The needle is then removed, and the sites of deposition are massaged to aid in dispersal of the local anesthetic. The procedure is repeated for the left internal

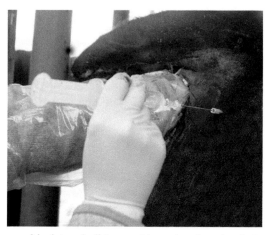

**Fig. 14.** Pudendal nerve block in a bull to provide regional analgesia to penis and prepuce.

pudendal nerve using either the right hand or some may prefer to use the same hand and rotate the hand to the opposite side.

The pudendal nerve block is helpful for examination and surgical procedures of the bull's penis in the standing animal including some teaser-bull procedures and to relieve chronic tenesmus associated with chronic vaginal prolapse in cows. Relaxation of the penis may take as long as 30 to 40 minutes for full effect. Effectiveness of the block may be assessed by firmly squeezing the tail of the epididymis of each testicle.[8] If the bull lacks the ability to retract the testicle in response to the stimulus this signals adequate analgesia. The internal pudendal nerve block lasts 2 to 4 hours.[32] To reduce the opportunity for the penile or preputial tissue to be injured following examination or surgery of the penis, the penis may be replaced within the sheath and the preputial orifice encircled with 1-inch adhesive tape to reduce the diameter of the orifice to aid in maintaining the penis inside the sheath until the anesthetic wears off. The tape should reduce the preputial orifice sufficiently so that the penis remains within the sheath but urine may egress from the preputial orifice. Once the local anesthesia has worn off the tape should be removed.[32–34]

## CLINICS CARE POINTS

---

- Evaluation of the penis and prepuce is critical to the validity of the bull breeding soundness evaluation.

- Dissection of penile warts located near the urethra should be carefully done in order to preserve future fertility.

- Performing a pudendal nerve block is necessary to provide adequate analgesia for resection of the prepuce when general anesthesia is not possible.

- Leaving an adequate length of prepuce (1.5 times the length of the free portion of the penis) when performing a preputial resection and anastomosis is critical to allow full extension post-operatively.

---

## DISCLOSURE

The author declares no conflicts of interest or sources of funding.

## REFERENCES

1. Carson RL, Hudson RS. Diseases of the penis and prepuce. In: Howard J, editor. *Current veterinary therapy: food animal practice*. 3rd edition. Saunder; 1993. p. 796–7.
2. Maxwell H. InabilitytoBreedDue toInjuryorAbnormalityof theExternalGenitaliaof Bulls. Bovine Reproduction 2021;155.
3. Carroll E, Aanes W, Ball L. Persistent penile frenulum in bulls. J Am Vet Med Assoc 1964;144:747–9.
4. Wolfe DF, Carson RL. Juvenile anomalies of the penis and prepuce: bulls. In: Wolfe DF, Moll HD, editors. Large animal urogenital surgery. 2nd edition. Baltimore: Williams & Wilkens; 1999. p. 233–6.
5. Ashdown R. Development of penis and sheath in the bull calf. J Agric Sci 1960; 54(3):348–52.
6. Ashdown R, Ricketts S, Wardley R. The fibrous architecture of the integumentary coverings of the bovine penis. J Anat 1968;103(Pt 3):567.

7. McEntee K. Fibropapillomas of the external genitalia of cattle. Cornell Vet 1950; 40(3):304–12.
8. Wolfe D, Beckett S, Carson R, et al. Acquired conditions of the penis and pre- puce. Large animal urogenital surgery 1998;237–72.
9. Wolfe DF. Restorative Surgery of the Penis. Bovine Reproduction 2014;155–71.
10. Anderson DE. Surgery of the prepuce and penis. Vet Clin Food Anim Pract 2008; 24(2):245–51.
11. Roberts S. Infertility in male animals in Veterinary obstetrics and genital diseases (Theriogenology). New Delhi: CBS pub and distri; 1971. p. 712–9.
12. Ashdown R, Coombs M. Spiral deviation of the bovine penis. Vet Rec 1967; 80(25):737–8.
13. Seidel G, Foote R. Motion picture analysis of ejaculation in the bull. Reproduction 1969;20(2):313–7.
14. Barth AD. Acquired abnormalities of the genital tract. Bull Breeding Soundness, 3rd edition, 2013, Western Canadian Association of Bovine Practitioners; Saska- toon, 145.
15. Ashdown R, Smith J. The anatomy of the corpus cavernosum penis of the bull and its relationship to spiral deviation of the penis. J Anat 1969;104(Pt 1):153.
16. Mobini S, Walker D, Crawley R. An experimental evaluation of the response of the bull penis to carbon fiber implants. Cornell Vet 1982;72(4):350–60.
17. DiFoggio AN, Prado TM, Yepez PRJ, et al. Theriogenology Question of the Month. J Am Vet Med Assoc 2021;259(9):991–4.
18. Walker D, Young S. The fascia lata implant technique for correcting bovine penile deviations. Mobile (AL): Society for Theriogenology; 1979. p. 99–102.
19. Wolfe D. Abnormalities of the bull–occurrence, diagnosis and treatment of abnor- malities of the bull, including structural soundness. Animal 2018;12(s1):s148–57.
20. Beckett S, Wolfe D. Anatomy of the penis, prepuce, and sheath, Large Animal Urogenital Surgery. 2nd edition. Baltimore: Williams and Wilkins; 1999. p. 201.
21. Lewis J, Walker D, Beckett S, et al. Blood pressure within the corpus cavernosum penis of the bull. Reproduction 1968;17(1):155–6.
22. Beckett SD, Reynolds TM, Walker DF, et al. Experimentally induced rupture of corpus cavernosum penis of the bull. Am J Vet Res 1974;35(6):765–7.
23. Wolfe D, Mysinger P, Hudson R, et al. Ventral rupture of the penile tunica albugi- nea and urethra distal to the sigmoid flexure in a bull. J Am Vet Med Assoc 1987; 190(10):1313–4.
24. Ashdown RR, Glossop CE. Impotence in the bull: (3) Rupture of the corpus cav- ernosum penis proximal to the sigmoid flexure. Vet Rec 1983;113(2):30–7.
25. Long SE, Hignett PG, Lee R. Preputial eversion in the bull: relationship to penile movement. Vet Rec 1970;86(7):192–4.
26. Long SE, Rodríguez Dubra C. Incidence and relative clinical significance of pre- putial eversion in bulls. Vet Rec 1972;91(7):165–9.
27. Venter HA, Maree C. Factors affecting prolapse of the prepuce in bulls. J S Afr Vet Assoc 1978;49(4):309–11.
28. Wolfe DFHR, Walker D. Common penile and preputial problems of bulls. Compend Continuing Educ Pract Vet 1983;5:447–56.
29. Desrochers A, St-Jean G, Anderson DE. Surgical management of preputial in- juries in bulls: 51 cases (1986-1994). Can Vet J 1995;36(9):553–6.
30. Hopper RM, Wolfe DF. Restorative Surgery of the Prepuce and Penis. Bovine Reproduction, 2nd edition 2021;210–29.
31. Sidelinger DR. Regional Anesthesia for Urogenital Procedures. Bovine Reproduc- tion, 2nd edition 2021;191–9.

32. Edmondson MA. Local, regional, and spinal anesthesia in ruminants. Veterinary Clinics: Food Animal Practice 2016;32(3):535–52.
33. Larson L. The internal pudendal (pudic) nerve block for anesthesia of the penis and relaxation of the retractor penis muscle. J Am Vet Med Assoc 1953;123(916):18–27.
34. Hopper R, King H, Walters K, et al. Management of urogenital injury and disease in the bull: the scrotum and its contents. Clinical Theriogenology 2012;4(3):332–8.

# Abnormalities of the Scrotum and Testes

Chance L. Armstrong, DVM, MS*, Aubrey N. Baird, DVM, MS[1]

## KEYWORDS

- Cryptorchidism • Inguinal hernia • Bulls • Unilateral castration

## KEY POINTS

- Cryptorchidism presents as a rare condition in the bovine but is widely considered heritable in certain breeds of cattle.
- Inguinal herniation is a cause of reduced reproductive performance in bulls due to disruption of thermoregulation.
- Indirect inguinal hernias are discovered commonly in young bulls that have been conditioned for sale and lose that condition after entering the breeding season.
- Direct inguinal hernias are a result of significant trauma and represent a true food animal emergency.
- Surgical intervention can salvage the reproductive potential of bulls presenting with inguinal herniation if there is not concurrent testicular damage.

## INTRODUCTION

The evaluation of the scrotum and its contents are part of the Bovine Breeding Soundness Evaluation (BBSE). The examiner should visually inspect and meticulously palpate the scrotum to discover abnormalities that could negatively affect the production, storage, and transport of spermatozoa. This would include a systemic approach that includes evaluation of the testicular parenchyma, epididymis, and spermatic cord. The practitioner should ensure that both testicles are present in the scrotum. Cryptorchidism is rare in bulls compared to species like the boar and the stallion.[1] The vaginal tunic surrounding the testes should be free of any fluid. The testes should be symmetric and a greater than 10% difference is considered abnormal. The tone of normal testes has been described by authors as having a meaty texture or that of a semi-flexed forearm of a human.[2] The scrotal neck is evaluated for presence of fat or swellings of the spermatic cords that could indicate a hydrocele or inguinal hernia (**Fig. 1**).

Auburn University College of Veterinary Medicine, 1500 Wire Road, Auburn, AL 36849, USA
[1] Co author.
* Corresponding author.
*E-mail address:* armstcl@auburn.edu

Vet Clin Food Anim 40 (2024) 69–79
https://doi.org/10.1016/j.cvfa.2023.09.003
0749-0720/24/© 2023 Elsevier Inc. All rights reserved.
vetfood.theclinics.com

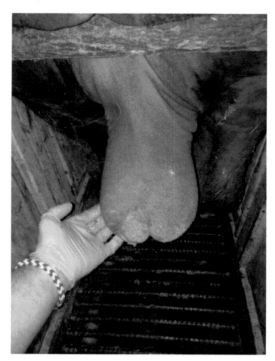

**Fig. 1.** Fat deposition in the neck of the scrotum.

The value of BBSE is compromised if the scrotal examination is not complete. The scrotum and its contents are best described to producers as being the sperm-making factory that also maintains a warehouse for storage. This factory must be cooled (ie, thermoregulated), or the quality of the product will be negatively affected. Practitioners may opt for diagnostics like ultrasonography and thermography when abnormalities are discovered upon palpation of the scrotum.

## EXAMINATION OF THE SCROTUM AND ITS CONTENTS

The scrotum and testes should be visually assessed as you begin your palpation of the scrotum, taking care to notice any outward abnormalities including swellings and areas of asymmetry. Palpation should be systematic in nature with the entire scrotum and all structures contained within it palpated carefully for abnormalities. The scrotum plays a vital role in the thermoregulation of the testes. The testes must be kept 4 to 6°C cooler than the core body temperature for proper function to occur.[3] Testicular thermoregulation is a multifactorial process that includes contraction of the tunica dartos within the scrotal wall to alter scrotal surface area in concert with the cremaster muscles to regulate the distance of the testicles from the ventral body wall. The scrotum is one of the few places in the bovine where sweat glands are found. Most of the heat exchange occurs at the pampiniform plexus that is positioned just proximal to the testicle within the spermatic cord. The pampiniform plexus is a dynamic intertwining structure consisting of the testicular artery and vein. The temperature of the arterial blood is cooled by counter-current heat exchange.[4]

Scrotal skin should be thin on palpation and free of any lesions that could cause thickening of the skin or impair the function of the tunica dartos such as frostbite or severe dermatologic conditions. Testicles should be freely movable within the scrotum with no adhesions between the scrotum and testes involving the parietal or visceral vaginal tunics. The amount of fat within the scrotum should be assessed, especially at the level of the scrotal neck. Large deposits of scrotal fat can lead to scrotal insulation and impairment of the thermoregulatory mechanisms of the testes. This condition is frequently encountered in young, over-conditioned bulls that are being fed for sale and bulls that have been enrolled in feed trials.

The entire length of both testicular cords should be palpated and should be smooth without any abnormalities such as inguinal hernias, abscesses, or varicoceles. The head or caput of the epididymis is palpated and can be found on the proximal anterolateral surface of the testes followed by the body or corpus of the epididymis which can palpated coursing down the medial side of the testis. The head is easily recognized as a flattened, U- shaped structure approximately 5 mm thick that is firmer than the testis. In order to palpate the body of the epididymis, one may push the contralateral testis cranially to allow for easier palpation of the corpus epididymis which blends into the tail or cauda epididymis located at the ventral pole of the testis. The corpus epididymis may be recognized as a band of tissue up to 1 cm wide and 3 to 4 mm thick.[2] Normal caput epididymides should be prominent and turgid, and differences in size and consistency may indicate an infection. Palpation of swollen, painful, indurated epididymal tail may indicate an epididymitis. There is considerable variation in the size of the caput epididymis and degree of adherence to the testis among bulls. Loose attachment of the epididymis to the testicle is occasionally seen. The significance of this finding is unclear but has been considered undesirable by some.

The practitioner should ensure that two testicles are present in the scrotum. Rarely, a bull will present with a single scrotal testis. True cryptorchidism, ectopic testis, complete aplasia of the testis and epididymis, or previous unilateral castration may all be differentials in these cases. In ruminants, ectopic testes are more likely to be encountered than retained testes because true cryptorchidism is rare in the bovid.[5] Ectopic testes are usually located outside of the normal path of testicular descent, with most ectopic testes being found in the groin region or in the pre-scrotal region along the prepuce and commonly only covered by skin and subcutaneous connective tissue.[1,6]

The entire surface of the testis should be evaluated for abnormalities and examined for symmetry, firmness, pain, and intratesticular or extra testicular swelling. The normal consistency of the testes should be turgid yet resilient palpating similar to a semi-flexed forearm of a human and is a subjective assessment of the testicular parenchyma and the enclosing tunics. If the testicle is soft this may be an indication of testicular degeneration as the seminiferous tubules may lack fluid and therefore normal spermatogenesis could be impaired. Progression of testicular degeneration can lead to a palpably excessively firm testicle that does not move freely within the scrotum.

There should not be more than 10% disparity in size between the two testes.[2] Once a disparity is noted one must make the decision whether one testis has undergone hyperplasia or if the contralateral testis has undergone degeneration or hypoplasia.

## CONDITIONS OF THE SCROTUM

Bulls suffering from scrotal or testicular disease or injury frequently have scrotal enlargement either unilateral or bilateral secondary to a variety of conditions. Visual and palpable information can be utilized to determine the source of the swelling and make a definitive diagnosis. The pursuit of additional diagnostics is warranted in some cases to further describe the extent of the cause and develop a prognosis for future fertility.

## Hydrocele and Hematocele

The most common cause of scrotal enlargement in the bull is fluid accumulation within the vaginal cavity which most commonly occurs secondary to trauma.[7] Fluid accumulation is usually unilateral but may be bilateral and usually secondary to periorchitis, hydrocele, or hematocele. Appreciable fluid accumulations are readily detectable by palpation of the testis (**Fig. 2**). The consistency of the fluid may be thin and easily displaced in the case of a hydrocele, or may be thicker as in the case of purulent material or clotted blood.[5] Ultrasound may be implemented to further characterize the nature of the fluid (**Fig. 3**). Hydroceles (accumulation of inflammatory exudate or transudate in the vaginal cavity) may occur unilaterally or bilaterally with the inciting cause yet to be elucidated. Several causes have been postulated including ascites, trauma, larval migration, high ambient temperatures, and neoplasms.[8] Hydroceles are commonly associated with decreased sperm quality consequent to impaired thermoregulation of the testes due to the insulation of the testes by the fluid. Spontaneous recovery has been reported in about 80% of cases within 4 months of diagnosis with return to normal sperm production.[8] Hematoceles (hemorrhage into the vaginal cavity) are commonly due trauma of the scrotum, testes, or pampiniform plexus with hemorrhage occurring directly into the vaginal cavity. Hematoceles may occur secondary to hemorrhage in the peritoneal cavity with movement into the vaginal cavity due to direct communication of the 2 structures. If trauma to the scrotum, testes, or pampiniform plexus occurs, the hematocele is usually unilateral with marked distention of the scrotum. Ultimately, the clot is resorbed followed by fibrosis and degeneration of the affected testis. Trauma severe enough to damage the tubular integrity of the testicle or epididymis may induce an auto-immune reaction due to extravasated haploid sperm inciting a granulomatous reaction.

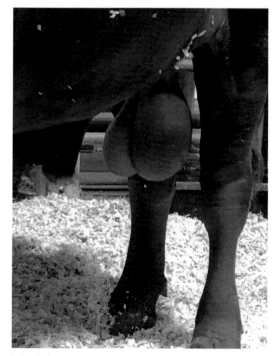

**Fig. 2.** Hydrocele of the left testicle causing unilateral scrotal enlargement.

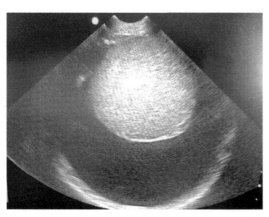

**Fig. 3.** Sonogram (7.5-MHz transducer) of a hydrocele with anechoic fluid in the vaginal cavity.

### Surgical repair of testicular conditions

Bulls with unilateral testicular defects such as testicular rupture, inguinal herniation, hydrocele, or severe periorchitis may return to normal testicular function following removal of the affected testicle. Confirmation of the unilateral nature of pathology is an important consideration prior to hemicastration. It is always a concern that the remaining testicle has undergone degeneration secondary to excess heat caused by any of the aforementioned conditions. The prognosis for future breeding soundness is dependent on the severity and chronicity of the condition. The longer the injury has occurred, the more likelihood the contralateral testicle has undergone permanent damage. It is the authors' opinion that semen should be collected to determine the health of the seemingly unaffected testicle. The spermiogram that displays copious amounts of head and midpiece abnormalities should be an indication that the other testicle may also be affected in cases where thermoregulation is chronically impaired. Bulls with such findings would have guarded future fertility. Implementing thermography and ultrasonographic evaluation can further define testicular disease or injury if available.[9,10] This is particularly important with bulls that have marginal value to the producer.

Unilateral castration is performed with the bull restrained in lateral recumbency and under heavy sedation or general anesthesia. The scrotum and spermatic cord are aseptically prepared and local analgesia should be provided with 2% lidocaine. Make a 15 to 20 cm vertical skin incision on the lateral aspect of the affected side that extends deep to but not incising the parietal vaginal tunic.[11] Blunt dissection is employed to free the testicle from the surrounding fascia. Sharp incision into the parietal tunic is required allowing exteriorization of the testicle and the spermatic cord for an open technique. Double ligation utilizing modified transfixing ligatures is recommend on the spermatic vein, artery, and cremaster muscles separately to avoid hemorrhage. Ligation of the cord and its contents with #2 polydioxanone suture is preferred by the authors. Some surgeons advocate for the use of an emasculator distal to the suture line to remove the affected testicle.[12] The excess vaginal tunic is resected and closed in an inverting pattern (eg, Cushing, Connell) over the end of the remaining pedicle. The subcutaneous tissues (tunica dartos muscle) and skin are closed after adequate hemostasis of the remaining pedicle (**Fig. 4**). In the authors' experience the cremaster muscle is the component of the cord that is most likely to hemorrhage. Extra care should be instituted to ensure hemostasis. Antimicrobials and nonsteroidal anti-inflammatory medications are administered for 7 days post-op. The bull should be evaluated closely for development of swelling during this time and BBSE should be performed 60 to 90 days following resolution of any inflammation detected in the post-operative period. Prior to unilateral orchiectomy, clients should be warned that a bull with one testicle, regardless of semen production following the procedure, will be graded unsatisfactory on a BBSE. Bulls that fully recover post-hemicastration will usually experience testicular hypertrophy in the remaining testicle and produce 1.5 times the amount of sperm that a single testicle will normally produce.[5] Retrospective data have reported 86% of bulls undergoing unilateral orchiectomy meet the minimum semen quality standards within 6 months of surgery.[13]

### Frostbite

Frostbite on the distal aspect of the scrotum is not an uncommon finding for practitioners in cold climates (**Fig. 5**). Providing dry bedding and wind breaks will help to minimize the risk, but despite best efforts some bulls will be still incur thermal damage to the wall of the distal scrotum from inclement winter weather patterns. Older bulls with more pendulous scrotums are more likely to be affected compared to 1 to 2-year-old bulls.[14] Frostbite results in scrotal inflammation impeding normal thermoregulatory functions of the scrotum and testes. Bulls suffering from mild scrotal frostbite often return to normal function with semen quality returning to satisfactory levels by late spring. However, cases of severe frostbite may require additional time for return of normal testicular function with normal function not returning until early summer. In some cases, damage to the scrotum may be so severe that permanent adhesion of the testes to the base of the scrotum occurs, permanently impeding the ability of the testes to move freely in the scrotum and completely hindering thermoregulatory mechanisms by elevating the testes close to the body wall.

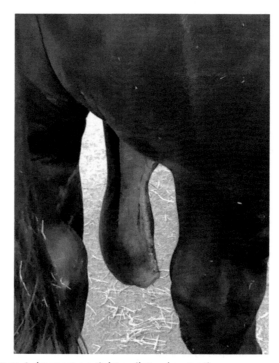

**Fig. 4.** Bull's scrotum 1 day post-op right unilateral castration.

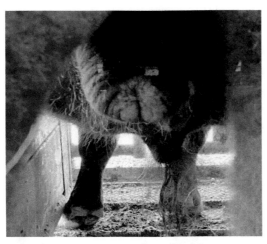

**Fig. 5.** Fibrosis of the distal scrotum as a sequela to frostbite.

## Dermatitis

Dermatitis of the scrotum can also be noted in some bulls especially in the Southern United States where hot, humid conditions exist. Nonspecific environmental conditions, bacteria, fungi, parasites, and scrotal sunburn or photosensitization in light-hidden bulls have been implicated as causes of dermatitis in the scrotum. Scrotal dermatitis has frequently been diagnosed in bulls housed in filthy conditions. *Stephanofilaria stilesi* has been reported to cause eosinophilic dermatitis. No matter the inciting cause, dermatitis often leads to thickening of the scrotum and impaired thermoregulation of the testes. Following resolution of the dermatitis, the scrotal thickness may return to normal. However, in severe cases permanent thickening of the scrotal wall may occur leading to persistent impairment of the thermoregulatory function of the scrotum.[15]

## Inguinal Hernia

Inguinal hernias may be diagnosed in mature bulls and can be classified as either indirect or direct. Inguinal hernias in mature bulls are not considered an inherited defect. Each type presents differently and poses different challenges for repair. An indirect inguinal hernia presents as a chronic condition that is not an emergency. The bull often presents on the complaint of hourglass shape to the scrotum due to the viscera entering the vaginal tunic in the neck of the scrotum. The anatomic narrowing of the vaginal tunics dorsal to the testicle is responsible for the characteristic shape (**Fig. 6**). The appearance of the hourglass shape may be constant or wax and wane as the viscera moves in and out of the tunic. The vast majority of indirect hernias occur on the left side and are attributed to the presence and weight of the rumen, as well as the tendency for adult animals to assume a right sternal position with the left rear leg abducted.[6] Bulls with enlarged inguinal ring were often extremely overconditioned at some point in their lives. During this period of overconditioning, retroperitoneal fat was deposited around the inguinal ring forming an inguinal fat pad and mechanically stretching the ring. As the bull returns to an appropriate body condition, the fat pad is lost but the inguinal ring remains enlarged. Indirect hernias are not considered a heritable condition but have been reported to occur more frequently in herefords and shorthorns.[16] During transrectal palpation, a dilated inguinal ring will be noted with viscera traversing through the inguinal ring. The rest of

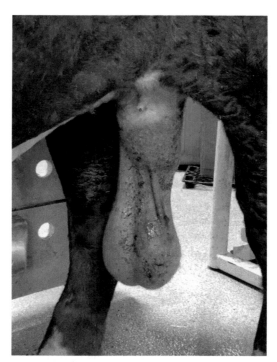

**Fig. 6.** Hourglass shape of a left-sided indirect inguinal hernia.

the physical examination is often unremarkable, and the bull presents with no clinical signs of gastrointestinal obstruction. Due to the presence of the viscera within the vaginal tunic, thermoregulation of the testes is altered and fertility impaired. Surgical repair designed to salvage both testicles has been advocated, but more often than not, the affected testicle does not return to normal function due to the chronicity of the altered thermoregulatory state. Therefore, it may be in the best interest of the bull and surgeon to remove the affected testicle during repair of the inguinal hernia. This offers the advantage to the surgeon that the ring can be securely closed to prevent reoccurrence without concerns of damaging the blood supply to the testis and possible hernia recurrence. The remaining testis will undergo hypertrophy and the bull can be expected to produce as much as 75% of normal sperm volume as he would have from two testes.[17]

Direct hernias result from a disruption of normal anatomy. This usually occurs at a weak area in the abdominal wall which in the case of the bull is the inguinal ring. The peritoneum in the region of the ring may be damaged and torn allowing herniation of viscera retroperitoneally through the inguinal ring into the space around the spermatic cord at the neck of the scrotum. Increased intraabdominal pressure is often implicated in these cases secondary to fighting with other bulls or athletic maneuvers like jumping impervious objects like gates or pipe fences. Intestinal incarceration is more common with direct hernias in comparison to indirect hernias. Trauma at the site of occurrence and the degree of swelling attending the herniation of viscera through the rent in the parietal peritoneum near or at the inguinal ring result in both intestinal obstruction and vascular compromise. The hourglass shape that is characteristic with indirect inguinal hernias is not present as the entire scrotum may be swollen due to the incarcerated bowel. These cases are a true emergency and bulls commonly display clinical signs of obstructive or ischemic bowel disease.[6]

### Surgical repair of indirect inguinal hernia

The standing flank and inguinal approach have both been described for elective repair of the indirect hernia. The standing approach offers the advantages of ease of restraint, animal positioning, and application for field implementation. The authors prefer the inguinal approach under heavy sedation or general anesthesia. This allows for better exposure and visualization of the ring and the contents that are herniated through it. The bull is restrained in lateral recumbency opposite to the hernia. The limb on the affected side is abducted to approximately 45° to allow for appropriate exposure of the external inguinal ring (**Fig. 7**). Make a 20 to 30-cm incision over the external inguinal ring that is in close proximity to the base of the scrotum.[6,16,18,19] Bluntly dissect through the fat and subcutaneous tissue to expose the tunica dartos muscle and sharply incise to expose the spermatic cord. The surgeon should reduce the hernia contents into the abdomen and consider the pathology to the affected testicle. Unilateral castration and complete closure of the ring could be performed if the surgeon questions the prognosis for normal function of the testicle or if recurrence of the hernia is a concern. The ring should be closed cranially if the affected testicle is to be salvaged to leave an approximate 3-cm (approximately 2 fingers) opening for the spermatic cord to traverse the ring. Heavy nonabsorbable suture material is utilized to partially close the ring in an interrupted pattern (simple interrupted or cruciate).[12,16] Antimicrobials and nonsteroidal anti-inflammatories should be administered for 7 days post-operatively. Hydrotherapy should be considered in those bulls that develop a significant amount of swelling after this procedure. Bulls have been shown to have adequate fertility following 90 to 120 days of strict sexual rest.[6,16]

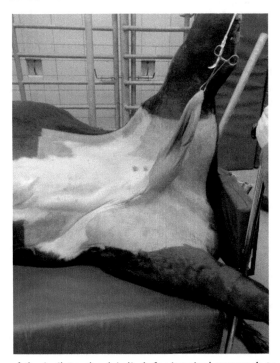

**Fig. 7.** Positioning of the ipsilateral pelvic limb for inguinal approach to herniorrhaphy.

## CLINICS CARE POINTS

- Ligation of each anatomical structure within the spermatic cord improves surgical outcomes following hemicastration.
- Evaluation of the ejaculate in the pre-workup of unilateral scrotal disease is important to determine the viability of the germinal epithelium of the contralateral testicle before surgery is considered.
- Hemicastration allows for secure closure of the external inguinal ring in cases of inguinal herniation.

## DISCLOSURE

The authors declare no conflicts of interest or sources of funding.

## REFERENCES

1. Jean GS, Gaughan E, Constable P. Cryptorchidism in North American cattle: breed predisposition and clinical findings. Theriogenology 1992;38(5):951–8.
2. Carson R, Powe T, Pugh D. Examination and special diagnostic procedures of the scrotum and testes. Large animal urogenital surgery. Baltimore: Williams & Wilkins; 1999. p. 277–80.
3. Waites G. Temperature regulation and the testis. Development, Anatomy, And Physiology 1970;241–79.
4. Senger P, TO P. Pathways to pregnancy and parturition. 3rd edition. Redmond (OR): Current Conceptions; 2012.
5. Wolfe DF. Surgery of the Scrotum and its Contents. Bovine Reproduction 2014;136–41.
6. Riddell G. Developmental anomalies of the scrotum and testes. Large animal urogenital surgery. Baltimore: Williams & Wilkins; 1999. p. 283–91.
7. Heath A, Purohit R, Powe T, et al. Anatomy of the scrotum, testes, epididymis and spermatic cord. In: Wolfe DF, Moll HD, editors. Large animal urogenital surgery. 2edition; 1998. p. 213–20.
8. Abbitt B, Fiske R, Craig T, et al. Scrotal hydrocele secondary to ascites in 28 bulls. J Am Vet Med Assoc 1995;207(6):753–6.
9. Purohit R, Hudson R, Riddell M, et al. Thermography of the bovine scrotum. Am J Vet Res 1985;46(11):2388–92.
10. Kastelic JP, Brito LF. Ultrasonography for monitoring reproductive function in the bull. Reprod Domest Anim 2012;47(Suppl 3):45–51.
11. Wolfe D. Unilateral castration for acquired conditions of the scrotum. *Large animal urogenital surgery.* Baltimore (MD): Williams and Wilkins; 1999. p. 313–20.
12. Ewoldt JM. Surgery of the Scrotum. Vet Clin Food Anim Pract 2008;24(2):253–66.
13. Ivany JM, Anderson DE, Ayars WH, et al. Diagnosis, surgical treatment, and performance after unilateral castration in breeding bulls: 21 cases (1989–1999). J Am Vet Med Assoc 2002;220(8):1198–202.
14. Barth AD, Waldner CL. Factors affecting breeding soundness classification of beef bulls examined at the Western College of Veterinary Medicine. Can Vet J 2002;43(4):274.
15. Brinsko SP, Blanchard TL, Varner DD. Male reproductive disorders. In: Smith BP, editor. Large animal internal medicine 4th edition, St. Louis: 2014, Elsevier Health Sciences, 1478.

16. Yepez PJ, Klabnik JL, Lozier JW, et al. Surgical management and outcome of acquired inguinal hernias in mature bulls: 13 cases (2005–2017). J Am Vet Med Assoc 2021;259(8):909–13.
17. Wolfe DF, Hudson RS, Carson RL, et al. Effect of unilateral orchiectomy on semen quality in bulls. J Am Vet Med Assoc 1985;186(12):1291–3.
18. St Jean G. Male reproductive surgery. Vet Clin Food Anim Pract 1995;11(1): 55–93.
19. Wolfe D, Rodning SP. Diagnosis and management of inguinal hernia in bulls, . Food Animal Practice. 5th edition. St. Louis: Elsevier; 2009. p. 356–9.

# Bovine Lameness from the Ground up

Gary D. Warner, DVM

## KEYWORDS

- Cattle lameness examination • Diseases of the hoof • Fracture repair
- Hoof trimming

## KEY POINTS

- Lesions in the hoof are the cause of up to 70% of all lameness observed in cattle. After a thorough visual examination, the lameness examination continues at the hoof.
- Subsolar abscesses, infected hoof cracks, and white line disease, when left untreated, may quickly involve the third phalanx on the distal interphalangeal joint because of a lack of soft tissue present in the hoof.
- Chronic subclinical laminitis resulting from subclinical acidosis is a life-long affliction, which can hamper cattle productivity and can have an impact on overall well-being.
- Pain due to injury or disease is the cause of lameness in cattle. Pain management, including medications and support bandaging, is a very important part of treatment and recovery in cattle.

## Introduction

Lameness in bulls is a common problem seen by many veterinarians, and the cause can be difficult to determine. Administering a proper lameness examination is particularly difficult in cattle due to their unique demands for restraint. Hoof testing, palpation of the limbs, and flexion and extension of the joints can be compromised by the method of restraint or lack thereof, and it can create a precarious situation for the veterinarian and support staff. Understanding cattle lameness requires experience and complete knowledge of their structural anatomy and handling. Access to proper facilities and equipment is important in getting an accurate result from the lameness examination. Unfortunately, financial constraints in place by the client often dictate what practitioners are able to offer. Additionally, some clinical diagnostic options available to other species are just not practical in bovine practice.

## EVALUATION
### Lameness Examination: Back to Basics

Every lameness examination should start with careful observation of the animal moving without excitation. If the problem is not obvious after visual examination, the next

Elgin Veterinary Hospital, 600 West Highway 290, Elgin, TX 78621, USA
*E-mail address:* elginbullvet@yahoo.com

Vet Clin Food Anim 40 (2024) 81–109
https://doi.org/10.1016/j.cvfa.2023.08.003
0749-0720/24/© 2023 Elsevier Inc. All rights reserved.
vetfood.theclinics.com

step is to properly restrain the patient on a hydraulic tilt table or tilt chute (**Figs. 1** and **2**). Casting is another option but it requires an abundance of labor and may not allow for an accurate examination because the amount of restraint required to keep the bull in lateral recumbency may interfere with his ability to respond to stimulation of painful areas (**Fig. 3**). Caution should be used in every case of restraint to avoid causing harm or creating a new injury.

Because approximately 70% of bovine lameness is in the hoof, the lameness examination should continue at the hoof. If hoof testing reveals a painful area, explore the area by paring the hoof and examine any cracks, crevices, or wall separations. If no response is evident on hoof testing, the sole should still be trimmed aggressively to check for a puncture, laceration, or developing crack that could lead to an abscess.

If no pain is elicited on hoof testing and no direct visual abnormalities are noted, continue the examination up the limb. Each joint should be palpated and individually flexed and extended, including the shoulder or hip. This can create a dangerous situation for support staff, and care should be taken to keep the limb partially restrained during examination but free enough to evaluate range of motion. Most often, lameness caused by a joint in the lower limb can be identified by flexion or extension of the joint, eliciting a painful withdrawal of the limb by the animal. The flexor and extensor tendons must be evaluated for sepsis or rupture. If the examination at this point has still not revealed the cause for the lameness, the practitioner should proceed with additional diagnostic measures.

### Advanced Diagnostics

Radiography, ultrasound, and arthrocentesis are useful in many cases of lameness (**Fig. 4**). However, if sedation is needed to safely perform these diagnostics, consideration should be taken to determine if other procedures, such as local anesthesia, would be inaccurate after sedation.

In the lameness examination, ultrasound is used to evaluate soft tissue injury of ligaments, menisci, and tendon sheaths. Arthrocentesis is used to make a diagnosis and prognosis when a joint is affected. Evaluation of cell types and protein level found within the synovial fluid is most important. Normal synovial fluid may include cell counts less than 1000 cells/μL and protein less than 2.5 g/dL. Synovial fluid from a septic joint would have more than 25,000 cells/μL and total protein of more than 4.5 g/dL.[1] Fluid analysis with values in between these ranges would indicate an inflamed joint.

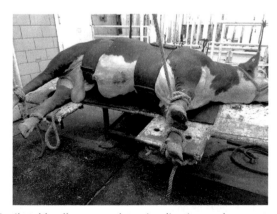

**Fig. 1.** A hydraulic tilt table allows complete visualization and access to the entire limb.

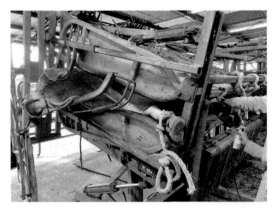

**Fig. 2.** Proper restraint in a tilt chute. Notice the down forelimb is tied to prevent movement.

## Local/Regional Anesthesia

The application of local anesthetics should only be done after physical examination of the affected area and all other available diagnostics have been performed. Lidocaine is used because of its rapid onset of action (3–5 minutes) and short duration (20–30 minutes). Standard preparation of the site for aseptic injection should always be followed.

Most often, the first site selected is vascular perfusion of all structures distal to and including the fetlock (**Fig. 5**). For regional limb perfusion, place a tourniquet (using IV

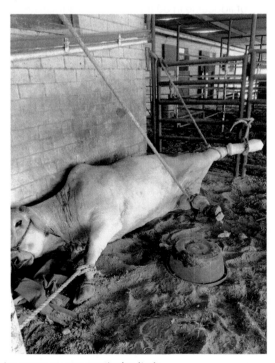

**Fig. 3.** Casting limits access to any particular limb.

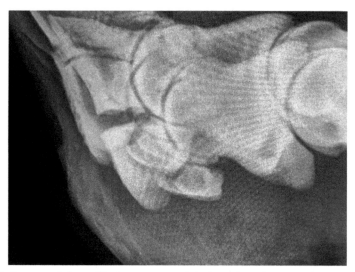

**Fig. 4.** This fracture of the coffin bone occurred during a breeding soundness examination.

tubing or bicycle inner tube) proximal to the fetlock. In a limb free of edema, wrap tightly enough to identify the dorsal digital vein and administer 15 to 25 mL of lidocaine. Maintain the tourniquet for 10 minutes before releasing the animal to observe for lameness. If no improvement in gait occurs, regional whole limb perfusion or a 4-point block may be used to isolate lameness below the elbow or stifle. To perfuse the whole limb, 30 mL of lidocaine in 50 mL of saline is administered with a tourniquet above the carpus or tarsus. This can be performed standing in a squeeze chute. The practitioner may also consider the use of intra-articular anesthesia for individual joints. Ten milliliters of lidocaine is sufficient for each joint except the stifle, which usually requires at least 25 mL in each of the femoropatellar joint and lateral pouch of the femorotibial joint.

In beef cattle with forelimb lameness, if the cause does not seem to be in the hoof, it is often in the shoulder and caused by inadvertent abduction during mounting or due to falls and displacement of the limb laterally. Rear limbs can be difficult to evaluate

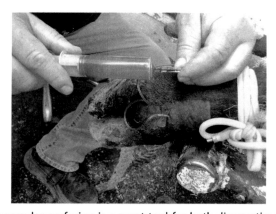

**Fig. 5.** Anesthetic vascular perfusion is a great tool for both diagnostics and treatment.

and require more patience and effort to examine. The coxofemoral joint must not be overlooked as a cause of lameness in the rear limb. These joints can also be injected with anesthetics to rule in or rule out lameness.

## CONDITIONS OF THE HOOF
### Laminitis

As stated, 70% of the lameness cases observed in cattle are associated with the hoof. Of these cases, 50% are associated with laminitis. Acute laminitis is caused by an acute metabolic or systemic illness and is characterized by reluctance to stand, arched back, and the appearance of "walking on eggshells." There are no outward lesions seen on the soles of the hoof, although inflammation may be observed in the coronary band and a digital pulse may be present.[2]

Subclinical or chronic laminitis is the more common form of laminitis and is due to periodic upsets in normal body function. Subclinical laminitis is not readily apparent at the time of insult but effects are compounded over time and become apparent weeks to months after the initial insult. The hoof flares out at the wall and has a flattened sole (**Fig. 6**). Closer examination can reveal white line separation with abscessation, vertical and horizontal wall fissures, heel erosion, and subsolar ulcers.[3] Horizontal lines (known as hardship lines) may be observed in a portion or the entire hoof wall (**Fig. 7**). Over time, more than one hoof can be affected. A few scenarios that can predispose a bull to chronic laminitis include the following:

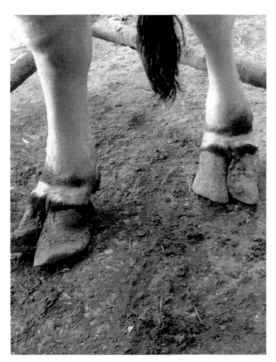

**Fig. 6.** This amount of hoof overgrowth is common in cattle after several episodes of subclinical laminitis.

- Nutritional mismanagement of the young growing calf
- Bulls on gain test
- Cattle being prepped for sale
- Cattle breeds involved with progressive genetic improvement/feeding trial
- Cattle being fitted for show

Because hoof overgrowth is the primary initiator of lameness, cattle with chronic laminitis should have regular hoof trimming to maintain proper hoof health.[4] The vascular damage that occurs during episodes of subclinical laminitis can lead to a cascade of hoof problems discussed in the following sections.[5]

### Solar Injuries

The metabolic effects of subclinical acidosis and laminitis can affect normal hoof growth and lead to white line separation, toe ulcers, heel erosion or ulceration, and sole ulceration. Puncture wounds and traumatic concussive injury are other contributing factors to subsolar abscess formation (**Fig. 8**).

Treatment of complicated subsolar abscesses and white line disease involves complete and total curettage of the overlying sole or hoof wall and removing all necrotic debris from the affected area.[6] Exploration of all tracts is necessary to evaluate the involvement of deeper structures (**Fig. 9**). If sepsis of the pedal bone or coffin joint is suspected, radiographs should be performed at this time (**Figs. 10** and **11**). Parenteral antibiotics and bandaging with antiseptic compounds should be incorporated into a treatment plan when possible. Although some practitioners elect to leave sole

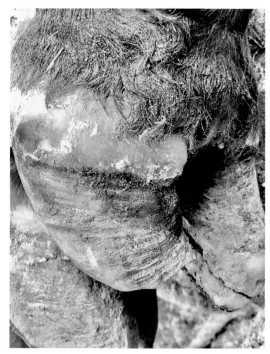

**Fig. 7.** Horizontal lines observed on this hoof wall are known as hardship lines. They are most often associated with episodes of laminitis.

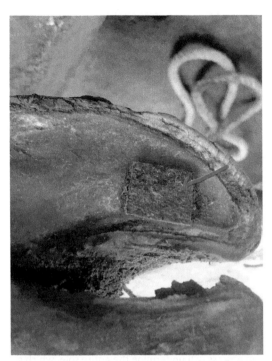

**Fig. 8.** Roofing nails are a common cause of lameness in cattle from suburban areas. Pointing to a roofing nail embedded in the solar serface of the claw (*red arrow*).

abscess lesions exposed, it is the author's opinion that these wounds heal better when protected. The application of a hoof block to the supporting claw prevents the affected claw from bearing weight and allows quicker healing due to the lack of contact with sole surface.

### Vertical Hoof Cracks

In a patient with a vertical hoof crack, lameness is caused by instability in the hoof wall as weight is shifted to the wall. Debris and soil may be packed into the crack. Remove all debris and necrotic tissue through careful curettage because any remaining diseased material can lead to sepsis of the laminae (**Figs. 12** and **13**). If debridement of the crack results in the penetration of the laminae, antibiotic bandages should be applied until the wound completely heals and the crack is dry and hard.

To stabilize a hoof crack, drill horizontally across the crack and place stainless steel wire across the defect in a bootlace pattern and apply an acrylic compound into the crack and around the wire. Alternatively, the crack can be filled with fiberglass cloth and acrylic compound or a quick-set urethane adhesive that allows direct application to the affected area without the need for any other material to support the repair. Stabilizing the crack will allow new hoof wall growth at the coronary band.

If there is radiographic evidence of abscessation or osteomyelitis, debride the area to allow for healing; curettage of the coffin bone and removal of bony fragments may be necessary. To alleviate pain during movement, apply a hoof block to the healthy claw or consider using a splint. Systemic antibiotics are always indicated in situations involving sepsis, and localized vascular perfusion can aid in increasing

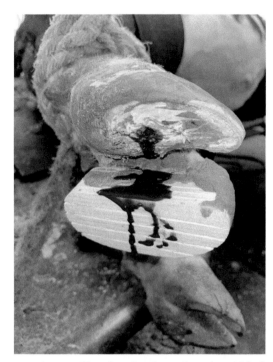

**Fig. 9.** In some cases, an abscess will undermine the entire sole, which should be removed to facilitate healing.

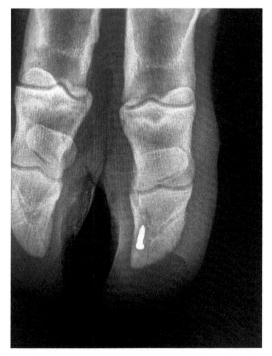

**Fig. 10.** Radiographs can be useful in isolating foreign bodies.

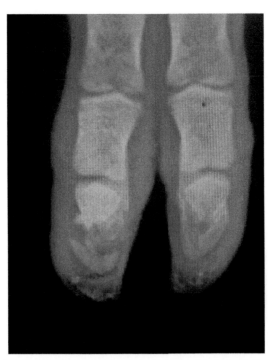

Fig. 11. Osteomyelitis of the third phalanx from chronic abscessation after a puncture wound.

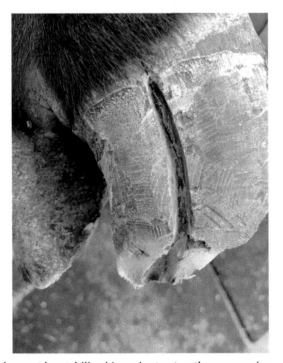

Fig. 12. Hoof cracks must be stabilized in order to stop the progression.

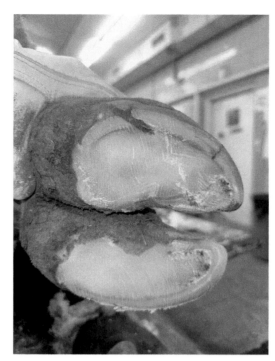

**Fig. 13.** Hoof cracks and white line disease secondary to subclinical laminitis.

antibiotic concentrations within the affected area. Potassium penicillin, ampicillin, and tulathromycin are commonly used for vascular perfusion. Medicated bandages, analgesics, and support bandaging of the contralateral limb should also be considered.

### Septic Arthritis of the Distal Interphalangeal Joint

Septic arthritis of the distal interphalangeal joint (DIP) is a common sequela to chronic infectious processes involving the hoof and/or interdigital space. Examination findings include a swollen coronary band with a draining tract occurring at the dorsal aspect of the extensor process, diffuse swelling of the pastern area, and partial or complete non–weight-bearing lameness. Radiographs will reveal osteomyelitis of the coffin joint and increased joint space with osteolysis of the second and third phalanx.

To anesthetize the hoof and provide postsurgical analgesia, perform regional limb perfusion using a long-acting local anesthetic, such as mepivacaine or bupivacaine. The following surgical approach to the DIP for arthrodesis is preferred over the abaxial approach because it allows better exposure of the joint.[7] Closely trim the sole and heel area and disinfect with surgical scrub and alcohol. Incise through the heel and deep flexor tendon to expose the intra-articular area between the navicular bone and the proximal extent of the caudal portion of the coffin bone (**Fig. 14**). It is recommended that the navicular bone be removed. A half-inch drill is used to facilitate curettage of the joint surface, drilling from the heel incision toward the extensor process and following the surface of the joint (**Fig. 15**). Debride all necrotic bone and use a squeeze bulb to lavage the surgical site with a broad-spectrum antibiotic or antiseptic saline solution. Place a wooden block on the healthy claw, pack the joint with gauze, and bandage the hoof.[8]

Parenteral antibiotics are administered daily, and bandage changes and joint lavage are performed every other day until granulation tissue has been formed. Beads of bone cement mixed with an antibiotic can be placed in the joint space to facilitate healing but they should not be placed until there is a healthy granulation bed and no more purulent discharge.

When the surgical wound has closed with granulation tissue, the limb is placed in a cast above the fetlock for 5 to 6 weeks. After the cast and hoof block are removed, the bull should be allowed a rest period. The lameness should show at least 80% improvement over the initial presentation; however, chronic mild lameness is expected.

### Corkscrew Claw

Corkscrew claw (CSC) is observed in the young adult beef animal and usually involves the lateral claw of both hind limbs. In some breeds, such as Brahman and their crosses, CSC can occur on the medial claw of both forelimbs (**Fig. 16**). Although CSC can be seen in calves and yearlings, it seems this is a management-induced problem rather than a heritable condition. Offering overabundant feed can lead to rapid skeletal growth and subsequent epiphysitis and angular and rotational limb deformity. This results in abnormal load bearing and compensatory changes in the hoof. To prevent structural changes to the phalanges secondary to CSC, corrective hoof trimming must occur during the active skeletal growth phase. In the mature bull, CSC cannot be cured, only managed.[2]

It is unknown whether bone remodeling in the distal phalanx is the cause or effect of CSC. In some patients with CSC, the second and third phalanges become

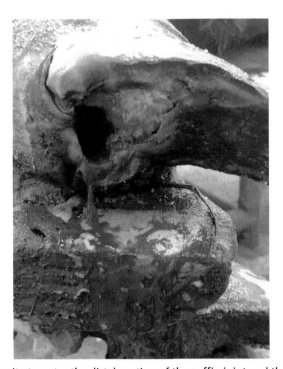

**Fig. 14.** Reference site to enter the distal portion of the coffin joint and the navicular bursa.

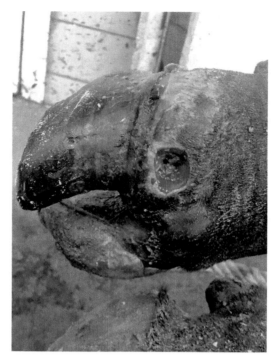

**Fig. 15.** Exit point for joint curettage of the coffin joint during facilitated ankylosis.

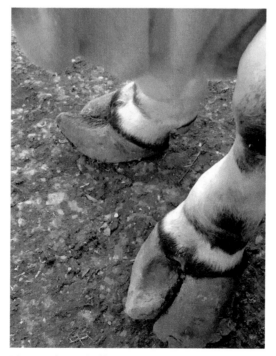

**Fig. 16.** Chronic CSC in a Brahman bull.

misaligned and the third phalanx becomes narrower with an abaxial curvature. This leads to abnormal load bearing, which affects the white line and leads to separation. In other patients with CSC, the growth rate of the middle to caudal portion of the wall is faster than the fore portion of the toe, which causes the animal to bear weight on the abaxial wall, predisposing to bruising, abscessation, and sole ulcers.

Correction of CSC involves balancing the weight-bearing surface of both claws. It is best to trim excess from the medial claw just until the white line is apparent. Next, shorten the affected claw to the same length as the normal claw. Remove the upward deviation and rotation of the wall with a grinder or nippers. The heel is often higher in the CSC, and it should not be lowered. Bevel the sole to encourage wall contact with the sole surface. At this point, there may not be very much area for bearing weight but it will encourage more favorable wear for the hoof wall.[6] Corrective hoof trimming should occur every 4 to 6 months.

### Interdigital Dermatitis, Digital Dermatitis, and Interdigital Pododermatitis

Interdigital dermatitis is a localized inflammatory process involving the interdigital space. In the early stages, the skin has a greasy appearance and some erosion can occur, particularly in the heel bulb area (**Fig. 17**). Digital dermatitis (hairy heel wart) is another low-grade inflammatory process with pronounced change when allowed to become chronic. The epidermal layer becomes proliferative, at first producing excessive hair growth that stands out from the skin and progressing to small papillary projections giving the appearance of wart-like growths.[9] These conditions respond well to treatment via foot bath but care should be taken in the choice of medications because some products may cause environmental contamination with improper disposal. A copper sulfate solution is considered environmentally safe.[10] In chronic lesions that are extremely proliferative, surgical resection and topical treatment may be necessary. The foot should also be bandaged with a broad-spectrum antibiotic or antiseptic solution.

Interdigital pododermatitis, commonly called foot rot, is an acute, aggressive infection that progresses rapidly (**Fig. 18**). Systemic antibiotics should always be administered in these patients in addition to bandaging.

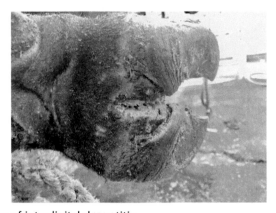

**Fig. 17.** Acute case of interdigital dermatitis.

## Interdigital Fibroma

The interdigital fibroma, or corn, is a condition most often observed in heavyweight beef breeds, particularly older bulls with widely placed claws (**Fig. 19**). If the condition is allowed to persist, the fibroma can become ulcerated and infected due to continued contact with the ground (**Figs. 20** and **21**). Local anesthesia and surgical removal is necessary to resolve the fibroma. Remove the prolapsed tissue and extract the fat pad (**Fig. 22**). Cautery of the vascular bed is sometimes required to control excessive hemorrhage. A bandage is applied with a sterile gauze and changed after 3 days. As an aid to healing, especially in the individual with splayed toes, it is helpful to wire the toes together to reduce swelling and decrease granulation bed formation. The second bandage can be removed in 4 days with complete healing expected within 10 days of surgery.

## CONDITIONS OF THE DISTAL LIMB

Lameness involving the distal limb usually has a traumatic origin. Most often, acute and severe lameness can be attributed to a severe concussive force, entanglement or entrapment of the lower limb within a fence or handling device, or foreign body penetration of the skin with invasion of deeper structures.

## Joint Sepsis

Joint sepsis often presents as severe lameness of several days duration that did not respond to broad-spectrum antibiotics administered by the owner. The animal will have an elevated heart rate and usually an elevated rectal temperature. Thorough examination should be performed under appropriate restraint, preferably on a hydraulic tilt table. The diagnosis is confirmed by obtaining a septic exudate on arthrocentesis (**Fig. 23**). Radiographs should be performed to rule out any concurrent fractures (**Fig. 24**).

Both systemic and local antibiotics via vascular perfusion should be administered. In severe cases, joint lavage must be considered though fibrin deposition seems to increase with subsequent flushes and can make joint lavage difficult. In cases that are slow to respond to treatment, arthrotomy or arthroscopic surgery may be required to remove fibrin deposits from the joint. Surgical drain placement is not advised due to

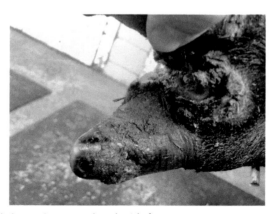

**Fig. 18.** Characteristic erosions associated with foot rot.

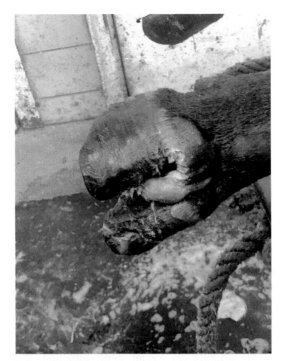

**Fig. 19.** Mature interdigital fibroma.

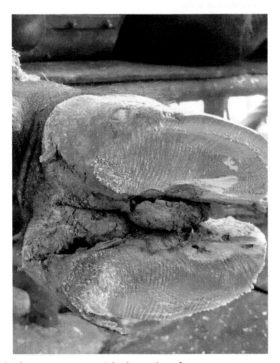

**Fig. 20.** This corn is close to contact with the soil surface.

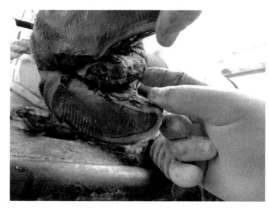

**Fig. 21.** Fibroma that has become ulcerated and infected. The fat pad is very inflamed.

the risk of contamination even with proper bandaging. Lavage can be incorporated with sterile bandaging to provide continued protection, although compression bandaging may suppress desired drainage.[11]

When there is marked reduction in exudate coming from surgical wounds, joint ankylosis can be performed after adequate curettage of the area by placing poly-methyl methacrylate beads impregnated with an appropriate antibiotic in the remaining joint space. When wounds no longer need attention, the limb should be immobilized with a cast and transfixation pins, as available. A support bandage should be applied to the contralateral limb.

### Tendon Sepsis

Sepsis of the superficial and/or deep digital flexor tendon is usually due to laceration of the caudal pastern or heel bulb area or extension of deep infection from a chronic hoof rot lesion (**Fig. 25**). A drain should be placed surgically from the pastern, through the tendon sheath and exiting above the dewclaw. Extensive lesions may require

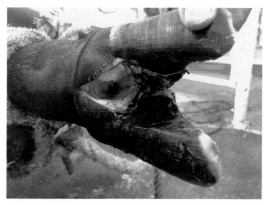

**Fig. 22.** Complete resection of the interdigital fat pad should be performed to avoid recurrence of the interdigital fibroma.

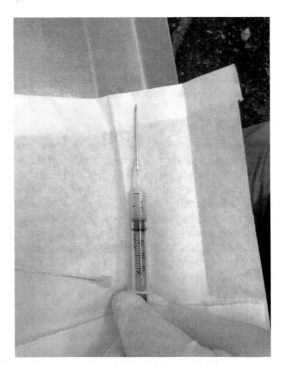

**Fig. 23.** Exudate from the tarsus of a yearling bull.

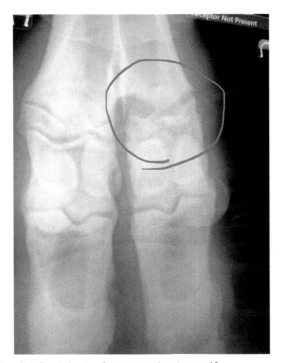

**Fig. 24.** Lysis of the distal epiphysis of metatarsal III in a calf.

complete resection of the superficial and deep flexor tendons (**Fig. 26**); this will require drain placement and packing with partial closure. Lavage may be provided in addition to frequent bandage changes, and the drain is removed within 7 days. Apply a hoof block to the nonaffected claw and cast the limb to the carpus or tarsus. After 4 weeks, the cast may be removed. Some deep digital flexor tendons may spontaneously rupture after treatment, which will predispose the patient to walk on the heel bulb.

## CONDITIONS OF THE PROXIMAL LIMB

Lameness involving the proximal limb is usually caused by traumatic events, such as during a bull fight, breeding incident, or by accident during restraint.

Suspected stifle injuries, including rupture of cruciate and collateral ligaments and menisci, should be addressed immediately, and treatment should be aimed at decreasing inflammation and reducing the development of degenerative joint disease (**Figs. 27** and **28**). Strict stall confinement is necessary for healing. Some injuries take up to 6 months to heal, and severe cranial cruciate or collateral ligament tears may require strict immobilization with a Thomas splint. These cases should be treated with long-term nonsteroidal anti-inflammatory drugs (NSAIDs). Of course, such injuries carry a guarded prognosis when considering return to breeding. If only the medial meniscus is involved, arthroscopic surgery may be of benefit in valuable individuals.[12] Long-acting steroids should be avoided because they may delay healing.

If stifle sepsis is confirmed with synovial fluid analysis, positive pressure joint lavage should be performed with a sterile isotonic fluid solution containing antibiotics and anti-inflammatories (**Fig. 29**). Follow-up therapies may include repeated lavage and regenerative medicine modalities such as plasma rich protein.

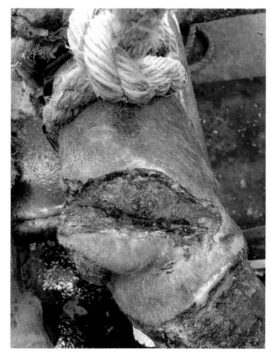

**Fig. 25.** Laceration of several days duration involving the digital flexor tendon sheath.

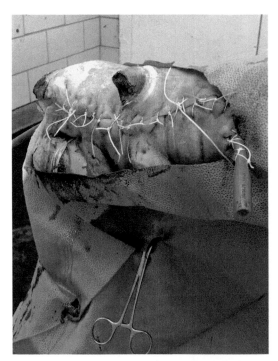

**Fig. 26.** Complete resection of the superficial and deep digital flexor tendons and their associated structure.

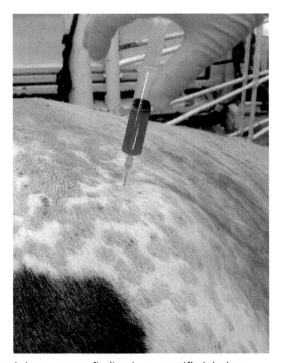

**Fig. 27.** Hemarthrosis is a common finding in many stifle injuries.

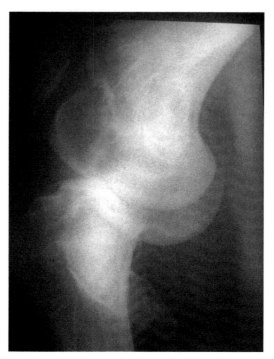

**Fig. 28.** This radiograph shows a stifle with complete rupture of the anterior cruciate ligament, which has a poor prognosis.

Non–weight-bearing lameness in the forelimb often indicates serious injury such as a fractured scapula or olecranon. A lesser degree of lameness may be observed with subchondral cysts (**Fig. 30**) or ligamentous injuries to supportive structures. Intra-articular anesthetics may temporarily improve lameness but rarely resolve all of the

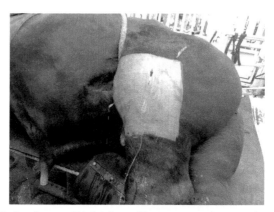

**Fig. 29.** Lavage of the femorotibial joint. This treatment is most beneficial in mild-to-moderate injuries and when performed soon after the injury occurs.

pain during examination. Treatment of these joints is usually relegated to the use of intra-articular injections and regenerative techniques unless surgical repair is financially feasible. For example, compression plating can be used to fix a fractured olecranon.

The carpus is probably the least affected large joint in beef cattle. Most lameness associated with this joint occurs in bucking bulls. Degenerative joint disease is observed in older bucking stock due to chronic hyperextension of the carpus when the bull "goes vertical." This condition responds fairly well to intra-articular injections of anti-inflammatories and the administration of NSAIDS.

## LONG BONE FRACTURES

Fractures of long bones often occur due to inappropriate management, such as mishandling, crowding, or improper handling facilities. After physical and lameness examinations, radiographs are necessary to determine if the fracture is comminuted or involves a joint. Attention should also be given to concurrent soft tissue injuries. Damage to the dermis may result in sloughing tissue and exposure of the fracture. Infected soft tissues can also lead to hematogenous spread of bacteria through the fractured bone.[13]

### Fractures of the Digits

Comminuted fractures of the digits usually require rigid immobilization in order to get adequate healing in a reasonable amount of time. Elevating the injured toe by

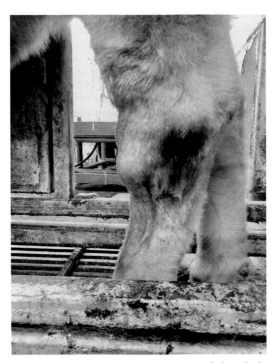

**Fig. 30.** Distention of the tibiotarsal joint secondary to a subchondral cyst.

application of a hoof block does not provide enough immobilization for proper fracture healing to occur, and many times, it will lead to a nonunion of the phalanx. A basic cast can provide sufficient support to restrict movement of the injured digit. Ideally, a trans-fixation pin cast (TPC) is used to provide solid immobilization of the injured digit, although this is not always financially feasible (**Fig. 31**). TPC is a form of external skel-etal fixation (ESF) that involves the placement of 2 or more transcortical pins through a bone proximal to the fracture site and incorporating those pins into a cast.[14] Wires are placed in the abaxial walls of the hoof to allow tension to be placed on the limb and are incorporated into the cast.[15]

For fractures of the digit, pins are usually placed in the lower to mid third of metacarpal or metatarsal III to provide for weight transfer to the cast. Predrilling of a slightly smaller hole (0.5 mm or less than the pin diameter) will reduce thermal injury to the bone during pin placement. Transcortical threaded pins are preferred to intramedullary pins in the mature adult because the transcortical threaded pin will be maintained for a longer period in the cortex before osteolysis renders it ineffective. Often times, only one pin is needed to properly provide for weight transfer in younger bulls. Two threaded transcortical pins are preferred in older or heavier bulls.

During cast placement, the pins are incorporated into the cast under tension with the pin ends cut even with the cast and topped with acrylic compound (**Fig. 32**). A "window" can be placed in the casting to allow for dermal wound treatment in com-pound fractures (**Fig. 33**). The cast should be removed as soon as possible to reduce the level of joint stiffness, generally in 4 to 8 weeks. If a bull becomes lame several weeks after the cast is applied, there may be an issue with the transcortical device, including fracture of the pin and/or osteomyelitis. If this occurs, the pin should be removed and the site lavaged. Antibiotics may be indicated. Occasionally a seques-trum may form within one or both cortices at the pin site; after aggressive curettage and lavage of the area, they often heal quickly.

### Fractures of the Cannon Bone

Fractures of metacarpal and metatarsal III respond very well to the use of TPC or ESF. In valuable individuals where cosmetic appearance is important, these methods pro-vides more complete immobilization and improved fracture healing along with better

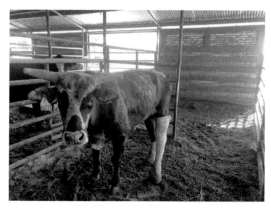

**Fig. 31.** Transfixation pin cast used to immobilize a compound fracture of metatarsal III.

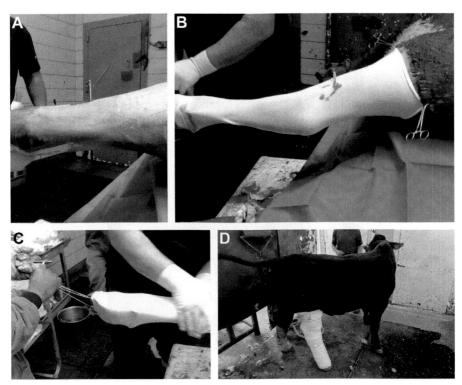

**Fig. 32.** (*A*) Proper placement of a transcortical pin. (*B*) Stockinette is placed over the pinned limb and is ready for cast padding and casting. (*C*) Wires are placed in the hoof wall to allow the practitioner to place traction on the bone and improve immobilization of the fracture. (*D*) Full limb cast. Care should be taken to ensure there is partial flexion of the hock.

overall alignment of the fracture fragments. Pins are placed across the cortex of the radius or tibia and the cast is placed as previously described.

### Fractures of the Tibia and Radius/Ulna

Special approaches are needed for fractures of the tibia and radius/ulna because external immobilization is difficult. Internal fixation with dynamic compression plates and screws should be considered in valuable bulls, although clinical outcomes are not always favorable due to implant failure and postoperative sepsis.[16] In animals of lower genetic or economic value, the modified Thomas splint and a cast can be used to immobilize the limb (**Figs. 34** and **35**). This system works well for fractures at or distal to the midshaft region and adapted as needed to allow for treatment of open wounds associated with the fracture.[17] This form of repair often works well in rough stock but these bulls need constant monitoring as fractious cattle can fall on the splinted limb and they may not be able to rise on their own.

The Walker splint is another versatile splint device used for immobilization of the entire limb and is particularly valuable in tibial or radial fractures involving the proximal one-third of the bone (**Fig. 36**). It is nearly always combined with casting of the distal limb. It provides lateral support by cradling the gluteal muscles and keeping the stifle

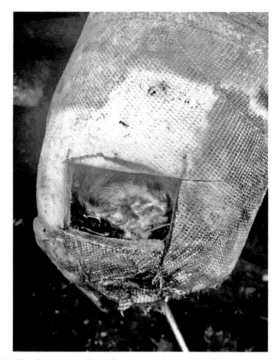

**Fig. 33.** Window in distal cast to allow for wound treatment.

and upper limb more upright as opposed to the abduction created with a Thomas splint, which can lead to further injury.

### Fractures of the Humerus and Femur

Fractures of the humerus can heal with strict stall rest if there is not significant damage to the radial nerve; however, the limb must be splinted to prevent tendon contracture.[18] Femoral fractures have a grave prognosis because attempts at repair have a high failure rate.

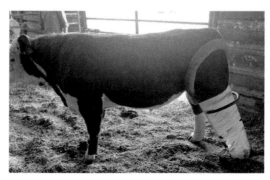

**Fig. 34.** Excellent positioning of this Thomas splint.

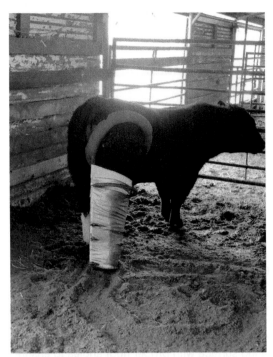

**Fig. 35.** It is extremely important that the "hoop" fit snugly on the upper hip/gluteal region to help give the bull leverage when he rises.

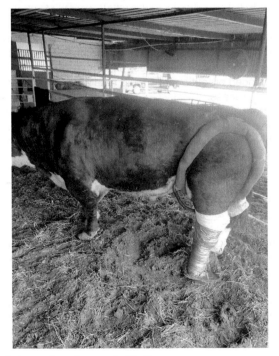

**Fig. 36.** Walker splint on a heavily muscled bull.

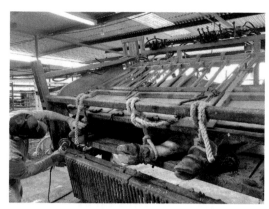

**Fig. 37.** Proper restrain in a tilt chute is necessary to reduce injury.

## HOOF TRIMMING FOR BEEF CATTLE

Hoof trimming services are a great practice builder. Much of the literature available discusses hoof trimming in dairy cows but the same basic principles can be applied to beef cattle. The Dutch 5-step hoof trimming method is a good protocol to follow; however, any method of hoof trimming will certainly work as long as the animal has an even weight-bearing surface with proper hoof angles to ensure balance and symmetry of the hooves.

Most beef cattle presented for hoof trimming have grossly overgrown hooves, often due to issues with subclinical acidosis and multiple events of subclinical laminitis during their development. After restraint of the individual, either in a hoof-trimming chute or in tilt table, the animal's hooves should be cleared of any excess organic debris (**Fig. 37**). Evaluate the length and angulation of the hoof and identify the amount of wall and sole to be removed. This process is almost automatic for the seasoned trimmer; less-experienced practitioners should take their time and assess all 4 hooves before beginning the process.

Starting with the front hooves, use hoof nippers on the lateral claw to shorten the toe to 3.25 to 3.5 inches. Proceed to trim the sole leaving approximately 0.25 inches of sole; when the white line is apparent, you have removed enough sole. As sole is removed, make sure that the remaining sole surface is level and even, front to back. Next, the medial claw is shortened and the solar surface is trimmed to match the lateral claw. When complete, both toes should be evaluated with a flat surface, such as a small board, to assure that both hooves are level.[19] Finally, the sole should be modeled, scooping the axial portion of the claw to create a dish-like effect on the sole, which reduces the opportunity for mud or manure to build up between the toes and gives a more natural appearance to the hoof.[20] After the claws have been properly shaped, address any solar defects and questionable wall areas (**Fig. 38**).

Once the front hooves have been taken care of, the rear claws can be assessed and approached in reverse order, starting with the medial claw. Completion of the procedure should be followed by overall visualization of all 4 hooves, paying particular attention to the interdigital space. If any evidence of disease is observed in this region, it should be addressed before removing the animal from restraints. The bull should also be examined as it leaves the trimming area to ensure he remains sound after hoof trimming and restraint.

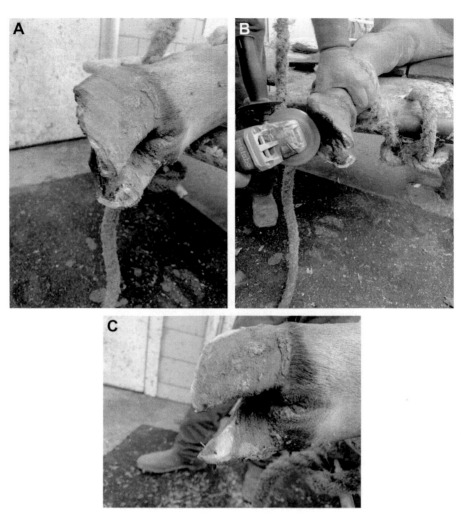

**Fig. 38.** (A) Start by evening the toes and excess wall with a hoof nipper. (B) Continue shaping the sole and wall using a power grinder with a cutting wheel. Friction discs are no longer appropriate and can cause excess thermal damage. (C) Desired hoof shape in beef cattle. Notice slight impingement on sensitive lamina.

## SUMMARY

Lameness evaluation and treatment can be a very rewarding portion of beef cattle practice. Even though economic decisions often play an important role in diagnostic and treatment plans, veterinarians can still work with clients to provide care for their patients at every scale of production.

## CLINICS CARE POINTS

- As 70% of all cattle lameness can be isolated to the hoof, it is imperative that proper restraint be available to thoroughly evaluate the hoof and its associated structures.

- Sepsis involving the hoof can spread quickly to deeper structures, including the distal interphalangeal joint and the digital flexor tendon sheath. Sepsis should be diagnosed and treated quickly and aggressively to avoid more serious problems.

- Stifle injuries in bulls are no longer a death sentence. Treatment options are available to extend the service life of a bull or allow time for genetic value to be preserved.

## DISCLOSURE

No disclosures.

## REFERENCES

1. Rohde C, Anderson DE, Desrochers A, et al. Synovial fluid analysis in cattle: a review of 130 cases. Vet Surg 2000;29(4):341–6.
2. Van Amstel SR, Shearer JK. Abnormalities of hoof growth and development. Vet Clin Food Anim Pract 2001;17(1):73–91.
3. Mulling C. Theories on the pathogenesis of white line disease- an anatomical perspective. Orlando, Florida: Meeting held on; 2002. p. 90–8.
4. Tarlton JW, Webster AJF. A biochemical and biomechanical basis for the pathogenesis of claw horn lesions. Orlando, Florida: Meeting held on; 2002. p. 395–8.
5. Hoblet KH, Weiss W. Metabolic hoof horn disease and claw horn disruption. Vet Clin Food Anim Pract 2001;17(1):111–27.
6. Shearer JK, Van Amstel SR, Brodersen BW. Clinical diagnosis of foot and leg lameness in cattle. Vet Clin Food Anim Pract 2012;28(3):535–56.
7. Greenbough PR. Sand cracks, horizontal fissures, and other conditions affecting the wall of the bovine claw. Vet Clin Food Anim Pract 2001;17(1):93–110.
8. Desrochers A, Saint-Jean G, Anderson DE. Use of facilitated ankylosis in the treatment of septic arthritis of the distal interphalangeal joint in cattle: 12 cases. J Am Vet Med Assoc 1995;206(12):1923–7.
9. Rodriguez-Lainz A, Hird DW, Carpenter TE, et al. Case-control study of papillomatous digital dermatitis in southern California dairy farms. Prev Vet Med 1996; 28(2):117–31.
10. Berry SL, Reed BA, Maas JP, et al. The efficacy of 5 topical spray treatments for control of papillomatous digital dermatitis in dairy herds. American Association of Bovine Practitioners Conference Proceedings; 1996. p. 188.
11. Verschooten F, De Moor A, Steenhaut M, et al. Surgical and conservative treatment of infectious arthritis in cattle. J Am Vet Med Assoc 1974;165(3):271–5.
12. Gaughan EM. Arthroscopy in Food Animal Practice. Vet Clin Food Anim Pract 1996;12(1):233–47.
13. Desrochers A. Diagnosis and Prognosis of Common Disorders Involving the Proximal Limb. Vet Clin Food Anim Pract 2017;33(2):251–70.
14. Lozier JW, Niehaus AJ, Muir A, et al. Short- and long-term success of transfixation pin casts used to stabilize long bone fractures in ruminants. Can Vet J 2018;59(6): 635–41.
15. Saint-Jean G, Clem MF, DeBowes RM. Transfixation pinning and casting of tibial fractures in calves: five cases. J Am Vet Med Assoc 1991;198(1):139–43.
16. Martens A, Steenhaut M, De Cupere C, et al. Conservative and surgical treatment of tibial fractures in cattle. Vet Rec 1998;143(1):12–6.

17. Anderson DE, Saint-Jean G, Vesweber JG, et al. Use of the Thomas splint and cast combination for stabilization of tibial fractures in cattle: 21 cases. Agri Pract 1994;15:16–23.
18. Saint-Jean G, Hull BL. Conservative treatment of a humeral fracture in a heifer. Can Vet J 1987;28(11):704–6.
19. Shearer JK, van Amstel SR. Functional and Corrective Claw Trimming. Vet Clin North Am: Food Anim Pract 2001;17(1):53–72.
20. Greenough PR, Vermunt JJ, McKinnon JJ, et al. Laminitis-like changes in the claws of feedlot cattle. Can Vet J 1990;31(3):202–8.

# Sexually Transmitted Diseases of Bulls

Check for updates

Arthur Lee Jones, DVM, MS

## KEYWORDS

• Venereal diseases • Bulls • Reproductive loss • Pregnancy • Abortion

## KEY POINTS

• Fertile bulls contribute to the reproductive efficiency of beef and dairy herds but also pose a risk of introducing or spreading infectious causes of reproductive failure.
• Practitioners are encouraged to consider diagnostic testing for reproductive pathogens when herd reproductive performance is unsatisfactory.
• An effective herd health process includes a biosecurity plan to reduce introduction of potential reproductive pathogens and control measures to mitigate spread of pathogens within animals in the herd(s).
• Although vaccinations are an essential component of a herd health plan, veterinarians are encouraged to perform a reproductive risk assessment in herds to determine possible hazards and exposures that threaten herd reproductive efficiency.

## INTRODUCTION

Reproduction is essential for successful cow-calf and dairy production and the most important economic trait for cow-calf producers.[1,2] For efficient reproduction to occur in beef herds, cows or heifers must conceive early during the breeding season, maintain the pregnancy, calve unassisted or with very little assistance, rebred in a timely manner and wean a calf every year.[1] In the case of dairy cattle, cows or heifers are expected to become pregnant, maintain the pregnancy, and calve every 12 to 15 months to produce milk. Interruption of that process leads to delay or total loss of production.

Pregnancy wastage or loss results in economic challenges for beef and dairy producers alike. Reproductive wastage can result from infectious and noninfectious causes.[3] Pregnancy wastage from infectious agents transmitted by bulls is a potential risk. In the United States, more than 97% of beef[4] herds and an estimated 25%[5] to 51%[6] of dairy herds breed cows by natural service.

Although fertile bulls are required to achieve reproduction, they come with potential risk of transmitting disease during breeding.[7] Pathogens that could potentially be transmitted by coitus include *Tritrichomonas foetus*, *Campylobacter fetus venerealis*,

Department of Population Health, UGA College of Veterinary Medicine, UGA TVDIL, 43 Brighton Road, Tifton, GA 31793, USA
*E-mail address:* leejones@uga.edu

Vet Clin Food Anim 40 (2024) 111–119
https://doi.org/10.1016/j.cvfa.2023.08.004
0749-0720/24/© 2023 Elsevier Inc. All rights reserved.

*Bovine herpesvirus 1, Bovine viral diarrhea virus, Leptospira* spp., *Histophilus somni, Ureaplasma diversum* as well as others not discussed here.[7] Some of these pathogens may not cause obvious clinical disease in the male or female but interfere with conception or result in pregnancy loss, often early in gestation.[8] As a result, producers may not be aware of possible reproductive problems until a higher than expected number of cattle are diagnosed nonpregnant or late bred at pregnancy diagnosis or do not calve when expected.

*Tritrichomonas foetus* and *C fetus venerealis* are classical venereal pathogens in cattle[8] requiring transmission through coitus or breeding with infected semen. Other pathogens may be acquired from the environment (*Leptospira* spp.) or transmitted through contact with other animals (bovine viral diarrhea virus [BVD] and bovine herpesvirus 1 [BHV-1]). The goal of this paper is to review sexually transmitted pathogens practitioners may potentially encounter in bulls.

## TRICHOMONIASIS

Trichomoniasis is a venereal disease in cattle caused by the protozoa, *T. foetus*. This single-celled, flagellated parasite colonizes the preputial folds of bulls who serve as asymptomatic carriers of the organism. "Trich" is endemic in many states in the United States[9] and is a significant cause of infertility and pregnancy wastage in beef herds in extensive range environments.[10] Cows are infected during breeding by an infected bull and bulls are infected by breeding an infected cow. In the cow, the disease typically results in transient infertility due to embryonic or early fetal death and abortion but occasionally causes pyometra or fetal maceration/mummification. Inoculation in the female tract during coitus does not interfere with conception or pregnancy establishment. The organism multiplies in the uterus and oviducts, resulting in endometritis and fetal death with abortion typically occurring 50 to 70 days of gestation.[8,11] Cows usually return to estrus 2 to 4 weeks after clearing the infection,[8] conceive, and successfully maintain pregnancy following resolution. Immunity is short lived and cows may be re-infected during the following breeding season.[8,11]

Chronically infected bulls show no apparent signs of infection. It has been reported that bulls over 3 years of age are more likely to become chronically infected, whereas bulls less than 3 years of age are less likely to develop a chronic state.[8–11] Presumably, this is because as bulls age, crypts or invaginations of the nonkeratinized, squamous epithelium of the glans penis and prepuce form which creates an ideal environment for *T foetus*.[8,9] However, others have reported no significant difference in number or area contained in epithelial folds (crypts) between older and younger bulls.[12]

Management practices that perpetuate this disease include introducing and/or keeping infected bulls or cows in the herd. A USDA NAHMS Beef 2007 to 2008 study reported that 53.3% of beef operations reported purchasing, leasing, or borrowing beef bulls 18 months or older or bulls no longer considered virgin with only 34.4% of the operations testing for *T foetus*.[13] In some cases, pregnant cows may carry the organism through gestation and be a source of infection after calving.[9] Real progress in controlling or eradicating the disease is hampered by the lack of knowledge of the true prevalence of the disease throughout the United States.[10] A 2004 report of beef herds in Florida found a herd prevalence of 11.1% (herds with a least one positive bull). However, a wide range of prevalence estimates have been reported in North America.[9] Differences in regional prevalence reports are attributed to regional differences in herd management practices, fluctuations in *T foetus* due to cyclic nature of the disease, and less than ideal sampling practices that may lead to lower detection of infected bulls.[9]

Only one report documenting the prevalence of *T foetus* in beef cows was found.[14] In that report, investigators tested samples from reproductive tracts of 503 cows at slaughter with real time PCR and detected *T. foetus* in seven (1.39%) of the samples.[14] Infertility due to infection with *T foetus* may be a significant cause of culling in beef cows.[9] However, due to the self-limiting nature of the disease[8] and low sensitivity of culture in cows, testing open cows for *T foetus* is not routinely performed on the farm.

### Control of Trichomoniasis

Testing bulls to determine if they are infected is essential for control. Testing bulls for *T foetus* is recommended for any diagnostic workup when investigating poor reproductive performance involving bulls. Surveillance testing is also strongly suggested during routine BSE examinations in herds in endemic areas.[11] Trichomoniasis should be considered in herds with poor reproductive performance with a history of exposure to nonvirgin bulls or in extensive pasture management where commingling with other cattle is possible.

Methods of collecting preputial smegma include preputial scraping with a dry pipette (most common and convenient),[9] preputial lavage, and penile sponge sampling with gauze. To collect a sample with a dry pipette, a syringe is attached to a rigid insemination or infusion pipette and inserted up the preputial opening to the fornix.[15] The penile and preputial mucosa is scraped vigorously, carefully avoiding trauma to the penis and contaminating the sample with blood. If possible, bulls should be sexually rested 1 to 2 weeks prior to sample collection to improve odds of recovering the organism from infected bulls[15] and reduce possibility of a false negative test.[11]

Sample handling depends on diagnostic test required. Samples can be examined directly for presence of organisms, cultured for 7 days in a commercially available culture pouch[a] or transported to a lab for polymerase chain reaction (PCR). Direct observation of the sample for organisms without culture is the least sensitive of the testing methods because the organism may be present in such low numbers as they may be missed. Culture improves the chances of identifying if *T foetus* organisms are present. Both approaches require the organism to be alive so careful sample handling is essential.[8,9,11] Laboratory PCR testing is done for official (regulatory requirements) testing or for diagnostic purposes and to confirm results of culture or direct observation. Some testing laboratories accept preputial washes/smegma or vaginal/cervical wash samples submitted in phosphate buffered saline, sterile saline, TF InPouchi, or TF transit tubes[b] for PCR testing. The PCR test can distinguish *T foetus* from other nonpathogenic trichomonads.[11] Many states accept a single PCR negative or "not detected" results for regulatory purposes and interstate movement.[9,11] Pooled PCR testing (up to 5 samples per test) is also acceptable as official tests in some states. However, if trichomoniasis is suspected in a group of bulls it is advised to test all bulls 3 times at 2 weeks intervals by culture and PCR to provide confidence that the bulls are indeed not infected.[9] Practitioners are encouraged to contact their diagnostic laboratory prior to collecting samples for advice on best collecting, handling, and shipping practices as well as test selection. A combination of culture and PCR testing along with serial testing reduces chances of a false negative test result (misdiagnosing an infected bull).[16]

---

[a] InPouch TF, BioMed Diagnostics, White City, OR.

[b] TF Transit Tube, Biomed Diagnostics, White City, OR.

In endemic regions, vaccination of the cow herd may be advised. The currently available vaccine does not prevent infection but it may reduce the chances of abortion[17] by reducing the time required to clear the infection as well as reduce shedding of the organism thereby possibly reducing the spread to noninfected bulls.[c] For optimal immunity, cows are vaccinated with an initial dose and given a booster dose 2 to 4 weeks later. The second dose should be administered at least 4 weeks prior to bull exposure.

Trichomoniasis is a reportable disease and there is no approved or proven treatment for infected bulls. All infected bulls should be sent to slaughter immediately.[11] Testing and regulations for interstate transportation of bulls vary by individual states and are updated regularly. Accredited veterinarians are advised to check specific requirements for each state prior to issuing Certificates of Veterinary Inspection.

## CAMPYLOBACTERIOSIS

Bovine genital campylobacteriosis, traditionally called "vibrio", is a venereal disease of cattle caused by the bacteria, *Campylobacter fetus* subspecies *venerealis* (Cfv). Clinical presentation for campylobacteriosis and "trich" are very similar,[3,8,15,18] and both should be considered when investigating causes of poor reproductive performance.[19] Like trichomoniasis, bulls are asymptomatic carriers of Cfv and effectively transmit Cfv during coitus to naïve cows.[18] Risk factors for introduction or perpetuation of the disease in herds is similar to that of trichomoniasis.[3,8,13,18,19]

The effects of campylobacteriosis are restricted to the reproductive tract and mainly observed in cows and heifers. Clinical signs are not observed in males and there are no changes in semen quality directly caused by Cfv. Cfv infection in cows results in a transient infertility, endometritis, embryonic or early fetal death and abortion, and possibly irregular estrous cycles.[8,18,20] Since abortion, with a few reported exceptions,[8] generally occurs in the late embryo or early fetal stage of gestation (less than 70 days),[8,20] the effects of Cfv may be undetected until pregnancy diagnosis or calving time. At pregnancy diagnosis, a wide range of gestational ages may be noted or a "bimodal" distribution of pregnancies observed with some cows bred at the beginning of the breeding season, then a large percentage of late bred cows.[8] Cows can develop a durable immunity to Cfv following clearance of the infection yet remain a source of infection for bulls until the bacteria are cleared from the vagina.[8]

## DIAGNOSIS OF CAMPYLOBACTERIOSIS

When low pregnancy rates or a bimodal pregnancy distribution is observed at pregnancy diagnosis, the practitioner will need to determine if the poor reproductive performance is due to infectious or noninfectious causes. The effects of venereal diseases may appear similar to other noninfectious causes such as poor nutrition or body condition and bull subfertility.[21,22] Because of the self-limiting nature of infections in cows, diagnostic testing usually begins with the bulls because there are fewer of them and since a thorough breeding soundness examination is an essential part of the diagnostic investigation, samples can be collected at the same time.

Prepuce samples for Cfv diagnostic testing can be collected by preputial scraping or penile sponge. If culture of the organism is planned, the samples must be handled very carefully, inoculated in a transport enhancement media, and shipped

---

[c] Trichguard, Boehringer Ingelheim, Duluth, GA.

to the laboratory specifically according to the laboratory instructions. Contacting the laboratory prior to sampling is essential. Culture of Cfv is challenging requiring support media and almost anaerobic culture conditions. The organism may not survive extended transport to the laboratory even in transport enrichment media. PCR testing may be a better test choice, as it is more sensitive compared to culture and does not require a live organism for testing.[21] If the bulls are not available, collection of vaginal or cervical mucous from affected cows or heifers may be useful.

## CONTROL OF CAMPYLOBACTERIOSIS

Vaccination is an effective management practice for controlling vibrio in cows and heifers. Cfv bacterin in oil adjuvants seems to be especially efficacious and provide longer duration of immunity than aluminum hydroxide adjuvant vaccines.[3,20,23,24] An effective vaccination program begins with heifers. Current recommendation for immunization includes primary dose of Cfv (can be included in multivalent, combination vaccines) with a second, booster dose given 4 to 6 weeks following the primary dose. The second dose should be at least 30 days prior to bull exposure. Annual booster prior to bull exposure is recommended. Vaccination stimulates a systemic humoral IgG response, whereas natural infection also produces a mucosal immune response in the uterus.[24] Vaccination immunization may not prevent vaginal infection. Although the infection may be cleared from the uterus, vaginal infection is still possible.[8]

Vaccination of bulls is also essential. Typically, bulls are vaccinated with the same antigens as the cows. Yearling bulls can be vaccinated with combination vaccines containing Cfv according to the same vaccination strategy recommended for heifers. Purchased bulls with an unknown vaccine history can be vaccinated during the quarantine period with the same 2 dose regimen.

Testing bulls is an important part of Cfv control. Especially when adding bulls with an unknown history or that have been exposed to other herds such as large public or communal grazing operation. Culling of Cfv positive bulls is recommended. However, carrier bulls may be treated by vaccinating with 2.5 times the label dose[d] twice with oil adjuvant vaccine and then annually thereafter. Bulls may still transmit Cfv after vaccination until the infection is cleared. Repeat testing is recommended to confirm bulls are no longer infected.

One 2013 case report describes dramatic reproductive failure attributed to Cfv in a beef herd in Saskatchewan, CN.[25] In the report, risk factors that complicated timely diagnosis and investigation of infectious causes of reproductive failure included bull injury, potential impact of semen quality following diagnosis of foot rot, limited bull-to-cow ratio due to bull injury, and failure to perform pregnancy diagnosis.[25] Testing for Cfv was not performed until the second year of poor reproductive performance after eliminating other possible causes. Practitioners are encouraged to consider Cfv when investigating causes of reproductive failure.

## PREVALENCE OF *CAMPYLOBACTER FETUS* SUBSP *VENEREALIS*

Much of the literature refers to Cfv as an important cause of pregnancy loss in cattle. In April 2023, Dr Hemant Naikare, Director of the University of Georgia Tifton Veterinary Diagnostic and Investigational Laboratory, Tifton, GA, sent an email to 35 veterinary diagnostic laboratories across North America asking if the labs had received any

---

[d] Vibrin, Zoetis, Parsippany-Troy Hills, NJ.

Cfv positive cases. Of the 5 responses, only 1 laboratory had a positive Cfv case within the last 5 years. The case was from an abortion panel performed on samples from a dairy cow that aborted in the last trimester. Cfv was not detected in follow-up samples from the bulls but the bulls tested were not the same ones that were exposed to the cow at the time of breeding (personal communication with laboratory personnel). Another laboratory reported 11 positive bovine samples in 2014 to 2018 but none since. Three reported no cases in more than 10 years. Although this informal inquiry is not a valid survey, it may be worth investigating if Cfv is still a significant reproductive pathogen in cattle in the United States.

Several reasons for few positive cases reported have been suggested: (1) sample handling and submission may have reduced the viability of organisms for culture; (2) not all labs use PCR for detection, (3) practitioners may not be submitting samples for surveillance or diagnosis, (4) use of vaccines has reduced the prevalence of Cfv in herds, (5) increased use of AI in dairies (some 100%) has reduced transmission, or (6) increased awareness of risks from nonvirgin bulls has reduce their demand and use.

Few prevalence studies have been published for Cfv in North America. One study from Western Canada reported a crude herd prevalence of 2.6% (2/78) and crude bull prevalence as 1.1%[19] in cow-calf herds in Western Canada. They also found that cows from herds that had a Cfv positive bull were 2.35 times more like to be diagnosed not pregnant than in herds with no Cfv positive bulls. According to the authors, the use of PCR as a screening test in low and medium risk herds may lead to false positives that in turn could result in culling of valuable bulls that are not in fact infected, costs of repeat testing to confirm, or increased costs of unnecessary control measures in uninfected herds.[19]

## OTHER POTENTIAL SEXUALLY TRANSMITTED DISEASE OF CATTLE

Although "trich" and "vibrio" are considered the classical venereal disease of cattle, bulls may transmit other pathogens during natural service.

*Ureaplasma diversum* is a common commensal organism inhabiting the reproductive tract of cattle.[8,26] It is also an opportunistic reproductive pathogen associated with granular vulvo-vaginitis, endometritis, abortion, and infertility in cows and heifers.[8,26] *Ureaplasma diversum* is commonly found in the reproductive tract of bulls and cows but is more prevalent in cows with various reproductive problems than fertile cows or heifers.[27] Cows and heifers may be infected during coitus by an infected bull resulting in vulvovaginitis, endometritis, infertility, or abortion at any stage of pregnancy.[26] *Ureaplasma diversum* transmission has also been associated with reusing intravaginal progesterone devices or contaminated applicators or other instruments.[26] Controlling potential iatrogenic transmission involves disinfecting equipment between animals, proper hygiene during reproductive examinations or treatments, and avoiding reusing intravaginal devices.

*Leptospira* spp. can also be transmitted through infected semen[7,8,20] and survives cryopreservation. Clinical disease caused by *Leptospira spp*. infection depends on the infecting serovar and host immunity.[28] *Leptospira borgpetersenii* serovar *Hardjo-bovis* is widespread in North America and is a significant cause of reproductive failure in beef and dairy herds causing abortion, infertility and weak or stillborn calves.[29] Infection with serovar Hardjo-bovis may lead to chronic renal carrier state and long-term urinary shedding.[28] In bulls, the organism can persist in seminal vesicles as well as kidneys and shed in semen.[20] Transmission of *Lepto* organism occurs directly and indirectly from the environment.[28] Persistently infected cattle shed organisms in urine and contaminate the environment. Warm, moist conditions provide a favorable environment for organism survival. *Lepto* organisms readily cross mucosal membranes such as the oral mucosa, gastrointestinal (GI) tract, and reproductive systems.[28] It is also zoonotic and can cause severe clinical disease in humans. Control measures include vaccination with serovar specific vaccines containing Hardjo bovis serovars and diagnostic testing and treatment or culling infected cows and bulls.

BVD and BHV-1, also referred to as infectious bovine rhinotracheitis, can also be transmitted through natural service by infected bulls. An excellent review of risk factors, diagnosis, and control for both viruses has been published.[30] Both are significant causes of reproductive loss and infertility in beef and dairy herds. Abortion and transient infertility have also been associated observed following vaccination with a modified live BHV-1 vaccine in naïve cows and heifers.[31] Although vaccination is also an important means of controlling reproductive losses associated with infectious agents, adhering to vaccine label recommendations is advised.

## PREVENTION AND CONTROL OF SEXUALLY TRANSMITTED DISEASE

Vaccines to stimulate immune resistance to the pathogens mentioned in this article are an important means of controlling reproductive losses. However, vaccines alone are not an effective strategy for control or prevention. Controlling introduction and exposure of potential pathogens, biosecurity, is the gold standard of disease prevention. Persistently infected cattle represent the major reservoir for pathogens that cause reproductive loss in herds. Ideally, limiting herd additions to virgin yearling bulls or heifers or pregnant heifers who were bred via artificial insemination should avoid risks associated with introducing reproductive pathogens from cows or bulls exposed to other herds.

Biosecurity and biocontainment are the first line of defense in preventing exposure to potential pathogens.[32] Quarantine of all herd additions and isolation of animals with clinical symptoms is recommended.[32] A good herd nutrition program and vaccination program are also essential to build resistance to disease resulting from exposure and infection. Surveillance, herd health and production records, and a diagnostic plan are also important components to respond to suspected reproductive losses associated with infectious pathogens. Herd owners are advised to build a strong relationship with a herd health veterinarian and develop an effective herd health program to avoid preventable losses due to disease or other causes.

## CLINICS CARE POINTS

- Reproductive disease are a significant threat to reproductive efficeincy in beef and dairy herds.
- The primary prevention of sexually transmitted disease is biosecurity and elimination of potential for exposure.
- Practitioners should be aware of means to prevent and diagnose reproductive diseases.

## DISCLOSURE

The author has nothing to disclose.

## REFERENCES

1. Funston R. Decreasing costs through improved heifer development strategies. Lincoln, NE: Proceedings, beef improvement federation; 2014.

2. Melton B. Attaching Economic Figures to Production Traits; 1995. http://animal. ifas.ufl.edu/beef_extension/bcsc/1995/docs/melton_traits.pdf.

3. Ball L, Dargatz DA, Cheney JM, et al. Control of Venereal Disease in Infected Herds. Vet Clin North Am Food Anim Pract 1987;3:561–74.

4. USDA. Beef 2017, "beef cow-calf management practices in the United States, 2017, report 1. Fort Collins, CO: USDA–APHIS–VS–CEAH–NAHMS; 2020. p. p45 #.782.0520.

5. De Vries A, Kaniyamattam K. A review of simulation analyses of economics and genetics for the use of in-vitro produced embryos and artificial insemination in dairy herds. Anim Reprod 2020;17(3):e20200020. https://doi.org/10.1590/1984-3143-AR2020-0020.

6. USDA. Dairy 2014, "dairy cattle management practices in the United States, 2014". Fort Collins: USDA–APHIS–VS–CEAH–NAHMS; 2016. p. p199. CO #692.0216.

7. Givens MD. Review: Risks of disease transmission through semen in cattle. Animal 2018;12(52):s165–71.

8. BonDurant RH. Venereal disease of cattle: natural history, diagnosis, and the role of vaccines in their control. Vet Clin North Amer Food Anim Pract 2005;21: 383–408.

9. Ondark JD. *Tritrichomonas foetus* prevention and control in cattle. Vet Clin Food Anim 2016;32:411–23.

10. Rae DO, Crews JE, Greiner EC, et al. Epidemiology of *Tritrichomonas foetus* in beef bull populations in Florida. Theriogenology 2004;61:605–18.

11. Estill CT, Schnuelle JG. Update on Trichomoniasis. Proceedings of the American Association of Bovine Practitioners, Louisville, KY, September 2020;24-26:313–6.

12. Strickland L, Wolfe D, Carson R, et al. Surface architectural anatomy of the penile and preputial epithelia of bulls. Clin Theriogenol 2011;61:362 (Abstract).

13. https://www.aphis.usda.gov/animal_health/nahms/beefcowcalf/downloads/ beef0708/Beef0708_is_BullMgmt_1.pdf. Accessed June 5, 2023.

14. Jones L, Palomares R, Rajeev S, Ensley D. The prevalence of Tritrichomonas foetus in cull cows at a southeastern abattoir. In: *American Association of Bovine Practitioners Conference Proceedings*. 2013. 201–201.

15. Thompson M. Infectious Agents: Trichomonas. In: Hopper RM, editor. Bovine reproduction. 1st edition. Ames, IA: John Wiley and Sons, Inc.; 2015. p. 524–7.

16. R Cobo E, Favetto PH, Lane VM, et al. Sensitivity and specificity of culture and PCR of smegma samples of bull experimentally infected with *Tritrichomonas foetus*. Theriogenology 2007;68:853–60.

17. Edmondson MA, Joiner KS, Spencer JA, et al. Impact of a killed Tritrichomonas foetus vaccine on clearance of the organism and subsequent fertility of heifers following experimental inoculation. Theriogenology 2017;90:245–51. https://doi. org/10.1016/j.theriogenology.2016.09.056.

18. Edmondson MA. Infectious Agents: Campylobacter. In: Hopper RM, editor. Bovine reproduction. first edition. Ames, IA: John Wiley and Sons, Inc.; 2015. p. 518–23.

19. Waldner CL, Parker S, Gesy KM, et al. Application of direct polymerase chain reaction assays for *Campylobacter fetus* subsp. *venerealis* and *Tritrichomonas foetus* to screen preputial samples from breeding bulls in cow-calf herds in western Canada. Can J Vet Res 2017;81:91–9.

20. Givens MD. A clinical, evidence-based approach to infectious causes of infertility in beef cattle. Theriogenology 2006;66:648–54.

21. Waldner CL, Garcia Guerre A. Cow attributes, herd management, and reproductive history events associated with the risk of nonpregnancy in cow-calf herds in Western Canada. Theriogenology 2013;79:1083–94. https://doi.org/10.1016/j.theriogenology.2013.02.004.
22. Vasquez LA, Ball L, Bennett BW, et al. Bovine genital campylobacteriosis (vibriosis): vaccination of experimentally infected bulls. Am J Vet Res 1983;44:1553–7.
23. Kendrick JW, Williams J, L Crenshaw G, et al. Fertility and immune reaction of heifers vaccinated with an adjuvanted Vibrio fetus vaccine. J AM Vet Med Assn 1971;158:1531–5.
24. Perino LJ, Rupp GP. Beef cow immunity and its influence on fetal and neonatal calf health. Bov Pract 1996;28:145–54.
25. Waldner C, Hendrick S, Chaban B, et al. Application of a new diagnostic approach to a bovine genital campylobacteriosis outbreak in a Saskatchewan beef herd. Can Vet J 2013;54:373–6.
26. B Crane M, Potter A. Re-evaluating *Ureaplasm diversum* and its potential role in bovine embryo transfer. Proceedings of the American Embryo Transfer Association 2018;98–105. Montreal, Quebec.
27. Machado VS, Oikonomou G, Bicalho MLS, et al. Investigation of postpartum dairy cows' uterine microbial diversity using metagenomics pyrosequencing of the 16S rRNA gene. Vet Micro 2012;159:460–9.
28. Grooms DL. Infectious Agents: Leptosporosis. In: Hopper RM, editor. Bovine reproduction. 1st edition. Ames, IA: John Wiley and Sons, Inc.; 2015. p. 529–32.
29. Wikse SE, Rogers GM, Ramachandran S, et al. Herd Prevalence and Risk Factors of Leptospira Infection in Beef Cow/calf Operations in the United States: *Leptospira borgpetersenii* serovar *hardjo*. Bov Pract 2007;41:15–23.
30. Newcomer BW, Givens D. Diagnosis and control of viral disease of reproductive importance. Infectious Bovine Rhinotracheitis and Bovine Viral Diarrhea. Vet Clin North Am FAP 2016;32:425–41.
31. Givens MD, Newcomer BW. Does modified-live viral vaccine administration to heifers or cows lack substantial risk?50 Omaha, NE: Proc / Am Assoc Bovine Pract; 2017. p. 43–8.
32. Huston C. Biosecurity and biocontainment for reproductive pathogens. In: Hopper RM, editor. Bovine reproduction. first edition. Ames, IA: John Wiley and Sons, Inc.; 2015. p. 259–66.

# Impact of the Sire on Pregnancy Loss

Ky G. Pohler, PhD*, Ramiro Vander Oliveira Filho, PhD

## KEYWORDS

• Sire • Pregnancy loss • Embryonic mortality • Fertility

## KEY POINTS

• Pregnancy loss during early embryonic development and late embryonic/early fetal development poses significant challenges in both beef and dairy operations.
• Numerous factors affecting sire fertility and inconsistencies in fertility evaluations increase the uncertainty of sire fertility predictions.
• Sires and the paternal genome have a major influence on placental development and pregnancy loss.
• Specific aspects of spermatogenesis seem to have lasting effects on pregnancy development and could be a reason for increased pregnancy loss.
• Estrus expression of the cow herd can also impact sire fertility and pregnancy loss.

## INTRODUCTION

Fertility is directly correlated with successful pregnancy and the generation of viable offspring. Livestock industries depend on prosperous females to remain economically efficient, but a female is not the only contributor to a pregnancy. In this review, we seek to further analyze parent-specific contributions to pregnancy outcome. The maternal and paternal genomes contribute differentially to mammalian embryogenesis, but both genetic contributions are required for a successful pregnancy. However, the precise mechanisms behind how each genome cooperatively interacts and generates a pregnancy have yet to be elucidated.

The phenomenon of pregnancy failure is conserved between species (humans, cattle, sheep, and others). This means that many species experience similar rates of pregnancy loss, making the comprehension of reproductive losses significantly important. For a livestock producer to maintain profitability, a common principle is shared to maximize the number of marketable offspring that are produced each year. However, the calf crop often yields below expectancy due to reproductive failure. Reproductive

Department of Animal Science, Pregnancy and Developmental Programming Area of Excellence, Texas A&M University, 2471 TAMU, College Station, TX 77843, USA
* Corresponding author.
*E-mail address:* Ky.Pohler@ag.tamu.edu

Vet Clin Food Anim 40 (2024) 121–129
https://doi.org/10.1016/j.cvfa.2023.08.006
0749-0720/24/© 2023 Elsevier Inc. All rights reserved.
vetfood.theclinics.com

failure is one of the greatest causes of economic loss in cattle,[1] and embryonic mortality is a primary contributor to this loss.[2] Embryonic mortality can occur early (< day 28) or late (day 28–60) during gestation (day 0 = estrus). If artificial insemination (AI) is done correctly, a 90% to 100% success rate in fertilization is expected in cattle; however, a significant proportion of those fertilized embryos undergo embryonic mortality by day 16.[2] Fertility studies are difficult to conduct and often require collection of the uterine tissues from slaughtered animals and subsequent uterine flushing. Thus, there is a limited availability of studies to analyze in this regard. Reese and colleagues[3] analyzed pregnancy loss outcomes through a meta-analysis from day 0 to day 7 of gestation (pre-blastocyst failures) and reported an average pregnancy loss of 28.4% by day 7 post-fertilization. Twenty-three percent of these losses were observed before day 4, suggesting that most failures may be due to issues in pre-blastocoel formation. Pregnancy loss emerges when there is impairment of the physiologic and/or genetic mechanisms that are essential for embryonic/fetal survival and development.[4] Contributions to embryonic/fetal mortality include genetic mutations,[5] uterine asynchrony,[6] failure in maternal recognition of pregnancy,[7] and impaired endometrial function that leads to deficiency in placental development.[8,9] The method of breeding employed also influences reproductive failure. According to a meta-analysis conducted in beef cattle, reproductive failure rates were found to be 32.2% for cows bred with AI following natural estrous expression, 49.5% for those bred with fixed time AI (FTAI), and 54.6% for those receiving an embryo through embryo transfer (ET).[3] Understanding the time in which reproductive failure is often seen can assist in understanding the physiologic and molecular mechanisms that cause embryonic mortality and this fundamental knowledge can be used to develop management strategies to decrease reproductive loss.

## PATERNAL CONTRIBUTION TO PREGNANCY LOSS

Fertility is dependent upon the male's and female's ability to yield successful pregnancies. Most studies, however, have focused on the maternal and environmental contributions to pregnancy. Few have focused on the sire and his role in pregnancy loss, and even fewer have elucidated prognostic relations between sire fertility and embryogenesis. This review seeks to analyze the male or sire-specific influences on other realms of embryogenesis in mammalian species. Useful tools to better understand these parental contributions are transcriptomic profiles, genome-wide association studies, and uniparental (parthenogenetic [PA] or androgenetic) embryos. There is increasing evidence that the sire contributes beyond early embryonic development, particularly to the development of a functional placenta, and recent findings (Pohler, unpublished) in cattle may point to the sire's genome having a more vital role in conceptus-endometrial attachment in ruminants than previously believed.

### Phenotypic Sperm Analysis and Fertility Assessment

Perhaps the most analyzed contributions of the male and his associated subfertility/sterility are defects in sperm. For sperm to successfully penetrate and fertilize an oocyte, they must complete capacitation, bind to the zona pellucida (ZP) of the oocyte, and undergo the acrosome reaction. These are challenging tasks, and impairments to sperm shape, movement, or chromosomal structure have been shown to negatively affect these events as well as the viability of a developing embryo. A commonly used estimate of male fertility is a visual inspection of sperm for abnormalities in a semen analysis. Nevertheless, the standard semen evaluation cannot account for the other functional, fertilizing capabilities of sperm.[10] More intensive parameters involve utilizing accessory sperm count, defined as the number of sperm that remain within the hardened ZP after mammalian fertilization,[11] and fertilization rate (FR). FR has been calculated as the ratio of cleaved embryos ~48 hours after in vitro fertilization (IVF) to the total number of oocytes exposed.[12] This technique is a useful tool for determining a sire's competency to fertilize an oocyte; however, FR is not an accurate depiction of fertility itself. A recent study reported nonsignificant differences in FRs of high and low-fertility bulls; however, the field fertility of accounted sires showed significant differences.[13] On the other hand, when assessing the accessory sperm count and the extent of development, the aforementioned high-fertility bulls had an increased number of accessory sperm as well as later stages of development in the embryos. An increased number of accessory sperm is positively related to fertilization and/or embryo quality, and later stages of development allude to developmental competency as well as the quality of an embryo.[11] This evidence suggests that competency to fertilize an oocyte is not a reliable indicator of fertility, as fertilization does not appear to be the issue at hand for these subfertile sires. The standard semen analysis, although useful for identifying most infertile individuals, has a profound shortcoming in identifying subfertile animals.

Meiosis is the process of creating haploid gametes, 4 daughter cells. In males, spermatogenesis takes place within the testes. Disrupted spermatogenesis can cause profound chromosomal abnormalities, in the form of meiotic errors, which likely lead to embryonic loss; however, these associations are seldom recorded in livestock species. In 2019,[10] a study was performed using 2 groups of human males with recurrent pregnancy loss: 1 group that had eventual pregnancy success through assisted reproductive technologies (fertile) and another that did not (infertile). All men showed a relatively normal semen analysis. Using Next Generation Sequencing to assess chromosomal defects, the results showed that both groups shared an increase in sperm aneuploidy, both in sex and autosomal chromosomes, as well as other genetic abnormalities.[10] Interestingly, Cheung and colleagues[10] reported the infertile group as having higher incidence of aneuploidy in sperm when compared to the fertile group of men. Moreover, the infertile group was capable of fertilizing oocytes that progressed to the implantation stage but ultimately resulted in loss. Therefore, these shared chromosomal defects suggest that recurrent embryonic mortality may be caused by spermatogenesis-related problems that are not identifiable through the standard semen analysis. Additionally, more profound errors in the haploid gamete may result in unsuccessful maternal-conceptus communication, ultimately leading to failed placental development. Therefore, impaired or otherwise altered spermatogenesis is likely associated with male subfertility or infertility and conserved across male mammalians.

## PLACENTATION

In eutherian mammals, the placenta is the most complex, specialized organ that will function as a multitude of the developing offspring's essential organs in utero.[14] Additionally, the placenta is a conceptus-derived structure responsible for nutrient exchange between the offspring and the dam, and it arises from trophoblast and extraembryonic endoderm cells in the early embryo. These are the first cells to undergo specification after fertilization; this is thought to occur because placental membrane establishment and functionality are critical in the earliest stages of pregnancy.[5] Without a placenta developing and functioning early, a pregnancy simply cannot continue. Recent work using uniparental embryos has begun to make headway on understanding parent-specific contribution to the placenta. In mice studies of uniparental embryos, the paternal genome showed significant contribution to the proliferation of trophoblast tissues which are placental precursor tissues.[15] The PA murine embryos, embryos which contain only maternal genetic contribution, showed relatively normal embryo proper growth and underdeveloped trophectoderm in the conceptus tissues. Opposingly, the androgenetic murine embryos, those that contain only paternal genetic contribution, had well-proliferated trophectoderm and an underdeveloped embryo proper.[15] These results provide evidence that the sire's role in a developing conceptus extends beyond fertilization; instead, the sire may be the primary contributor to functional placental development. Moreover, preliminary data (Pohler, unpublished) using PA bovine embryos may extend this narrative to other placenta types. Ruminants and other livestock species utilize a synepitheliochorial placenta whereas rodents and humans have a hemochorial placenta. The ET of bovine PAs allowed for in vivo comparisons against biparental pregnancies. The results showed significant differentially expressed genes (DEGs) of PAs versus control bovine pregnancies. Of those DEGs, PAs showed decreases in genes critical for the maintenance of pregnancy. These included structural activities, reduction-oxidation reactions, and proteolytic activities involving pregnancy-associated glycoproteins (PAGs). Interestingly, at day 31, the trophectoderm of the PA pregnancies was well-elongated, but it was rudimentary in nature and had no obvious sites of attachment. This further suggests that the maternal versus paternal role in the developing conceptus is different and infers a potential role of the sire beyond simply forming a placenta. Instead, the paternal genome may be intricately involved in attachment and perhaps the implantation process in bovine pregnancies. Chimera ET studies (aggregates of in vitro and PA blastocysts) in cattle may further support the idea that the sire's genome plays a strong role in the full development of extraembryonic, placental structures as well as a viable calf.[16] Where bovine, uniparental PA pregnancies ultimately failed, the combination of in vitro–derived, biparental blastomeres with PA blastomeres led to live-birth chimeric calves.[16] Additionally, Boediono and colleagues[16] hypothesized that the IVF blastomeres would allocate to the trophectoderm while the PA blastomeres would give rise to the inner cell mass, thus shedding light on the paternal genome's necessity in placental tissues, but no substantiating evidence has arisen since.

### Placenta-Specific Molecules

In addition to functioning as vital organs to a developing conceptus, the placenta, of predominantly paternal origin, also contributes its own products to promote pregnancy maintenance. These classes of pregnancy-specific molecules are produced by the trophoblast giant cells of the placenta and are secreted into the maternal circulation during pregnancy.[17,18] In cattle, PAGs are abundantly expressed in maternal circulation. Since their discovery in the 1980s, PAGs have been a target for pregnancy diagnosis and prediction of pregnancy loss. In cattle, relative PAG concentrations are commercially used to detect pregnancies, and they are indicative markers of late embryonic mortality which comprises approximately 6% of bovine pregnancy loss.[3] In bovine pregnancies with relatively high peripheral PAG concentrations, embryonic survival was increased as compared to those with lower concentrations.[8,19–22] Moreover, in these studies sires were randomized and identified as either high or low–pregnancy loss sires. Interestingly, the pregnancies by low-fertility (increased pregnancy loss) sires had lower circulating PAG concentration compared to high-fertility sired pregnancies. These experiments together provide solid evidence that low-fertility (high pregnancy loss) bulls influence PAG production and exhibit variability at the PAG locus contributing to pregnancy loss. Reasons behind why individual sires have shown higher incidences of pregnancy loss remain under investigation, but it is suggested that differences in PAG expression or translation to maternal circulation (via placental development) may be a major component behind these losses.

### Genetic and Transcriptomic Factors

Moreover, sires bring more than just the paternal half of the genome to an oocyte; sperm have been found to also carry RNA transcripts and associated proteins. These transcripts may be either intact or fragmented but are believed to play a role in early pregnancy. In 2017, a study by Selvaraju and colleagues[23] reported a novel, full transcriptomic profile of fresh bovine semen. Among the transcripts identified, Selvaraju and colleagues[23] observed many that were significantly associated with fertilization events and embryogenesis. Furthermore, in this study 16 of the PAG proteins were identified as intact RNA transcripts, with high abundance in sperm. Among the transcripts with the highest abundance were *THSD4* and *PAG5*, both of which have strong associations with placental development.[23] Given the sampling took place with known fertile bulls and considering the previous findings regarding high–pregnancy loss sires,[22,24] it is reasonable to suggest that these paternal-origin PAG transcripts, among others, may have a significant role in the pregnancy outcome. These factors, however, cannot be detected by standard semen evaluations. Although it is strongly suggested, beyond zygotic genome activation, no investigational evidence exists as to whether these transcripts are directly involved in embryonic development itself.[23]

### Genomic Imprinting

The parental genomes must work in tandem to successfully generate a pregnancy, but each parent's set of genes does not behave the same in a developing conceptus. In placental mammals, genomic imprinting is a phenomenon thought to have arisen to "silence" opposing parental alleles in situations where biallelic expression could lead to developmental errors or lethality. There are 2 rounds of imprinting that occur. The first of which occurs at fertilization (first-generation imprints) and is maintained throughout the individual's lifetime, but erasure and reprogramming occur in the gonads of that individual in utero (second-generation imprints), determined by the offspring's gender.[25–28] Most identified genetic imprints have been associated with embryogenesis, and most of those identified in cattle and other species are within the placenta, a vital prenatal organ of strong paternal influence.[15,29] Therefore, if failure or other errors occur during genomic imprinting in the gametes of an individual, detrimental consequences are likely to result (**Fig. 1**).

While inspecting rodent PA conceptuses, studies in 1984 observed abnormal embryos and growth-retarded–associated placental structures.[15,29] Failure in this critical stage is not typically permissive by nature since most, if not all, failed first-generation genomic imprints are thought to be associated with developmental errors and lethality.[26] Thus, it is reasonable to suggest that prenatal failure regarding genomic imprinting in the male may be a causative factor in embryonic mortality in cattle and other placental mammals. The parental genomes are nonequivalent; both must play pivotal, individual roles in the natural generation of offspring. The paternal genome must be present and successfully imprinted to ensure critical developmental steps can occur. Otherwise, embryonic loss is likely the outcome. The importance of the paternal genome is often overlooked, underappreciated, and underestimated. This has led to underwhelming information regarding the paternal role in a successful pregnancy. Moreover, there is stark limited information regarding imprinted genes in livestock species. At present, $\sim$274 imprinted genes have been identified in humans and $\sim$178 in mice, while only $\sim$50 and $\sim$31 have been identified in cattle and sheep,

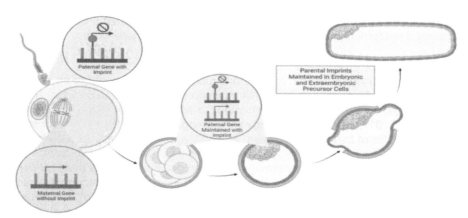

**Fig. 1.** First-generation genomic imprints in early embryos and parentally derived developmental structures. The figure above shows an example of a first-generation paternally imprinted gene. At fertilization, the sperm contributes a haploid set of chromosomes with the indicated imprinted gene, and the same gene within the oocyte is not imprinted. The resulting zygote retains this paternally imprinted status in said gene and, thus, only expresses the maternal version of the gene. The ICM, shaded in yellow, gives rise to maternally derived embryogenesis products while EE and TB, shaded above in light and dark blue, give rise to paternally derived embryogenesis products. Eventually, the ICM will form the embryo proper while the EE and TB will form the associated placental membranes. EE, extraembryonic endoderm; ICM, inner cell mass; TB, trophoblast.

respectively. With increasing evidence of parent-specific roles at a genetic level in mammalian species, more attention should be directed toward the paternal genome to better understand the sire's contribution to conceptus development and loss.

## SIRE FIELD FERTILITY

Estrus expression near the time of FTAI is correlated with pregnancy success due to positive impacts on ovarian function and the uterine environment, which affect embryo development and pregnancy maintenance.[8,21,30,31] Pre-ovulatory estradiol associated with estrus expression directly affects pregnancy establishment and maintenance through several physiologic events including gamete transport and preparation of the uterine environment.[30,32–34] Franco and colleagues[22,24] tested whether pregnancy rates differ among sires when cows either expressed estrus before FTAI or did not and observed that a large variation existed among sires. For example, cows inseminated with semen from one sire had a 50% increase in pregnancy rate at day 30 when they expressed estrus before or at the time of FTAI, whereas cows inseminated with semen from a different sire experienced only a 4% increase in pregnancy rate. Multiple studies have reported similar effects of estrus expression and pregnancy loss in both beef and dairy cattle.[22,24,30] Studies have reported that changes in the uterine environment, including changes in pH following estrus expression, affect sperm transport and longevity.[35] These changes contribute to an enhanced sperm viability until the time of ovulation. Even though there is not a clear reason for this variation among sires, the aforementioned discussion regarding sperm characteristics (genetic or molecular) may explain why certain sires seem to be more resilient to changes in the uterine environment compared to others. This resilience may be associated, at least in part, with variations in sperm longevity.

## SUMMARY

Prediction of male fertility remains elusive. Developing in vitro techniques to accurately predict field fertility would have a major impact on increasing overall reproductive efficiency. It is important to realize that even when sperm appear to possess all the required traits for successful fertilization, relative differences still exist, emphasizing the need for a better understanding of the molecular and genetic components of sperm, as well as the interaction between sperm and the female reproductive tract following insemination. Another key point is that sires have a significant contribution to pregnancy loss, which should not be disregarded when assessing fertility. Exploring these interactions can help us understand the causes of pregnancy loss, as well as develop tools to identify and select higher fertility sires.

## DISCLOSURE

Authors have no disclosure.

## FUNDING

This project was supported by Agriculture and Food Research Initiative Competitive Grant no. 2019-67015-28998 from USDA NIFA.

## REFERENCES

1. Bellows D, Ott S, Bellows R. Cost of reproductive diseases and conditions in cattle. The Professional Animal Scientist 2002;18:26–32.
2. Diskin MG, Morris DG. Embryonic and Early Foetal Losses in Cattle and Other Ruminants. Reprod Domest Anim 2008;43:260–7.
3. Reese S, Franco G, Poole R, et al. Pregnancy loss in beef cattle: A meta-analysis. Anim Reprod Sci 2020;212:106251.
4. Farin PW, Piedrahita JA, Farin CE. Errors in development of fetuses and placentas from in vitro-produced bovine embryos. Theriogenology 2006;65:178–91.
5. Cross JC. Formation of the placenta and extraembryonic membranes. Ann N Y Acad Sci 1998;857:23–32.
6. Pope WF. Uterine asynchrony: a cause of embryonic loss. Biol Reprod 1988;39: 999–1003.
7. Cheng Z, Abudureyimu A, Oguejiofor CF, et al. BVDV alters uterine prostaglandin production during pregnancy recognition in cows. Reproduction 2016;151.
8. Pohler KG, Pereira MHC, Lopes FR, et al. Circulating concentrations of bovine pregnancy-associated glycoproteins and late embryonic mortality in lactating dairy herds. J Dairy Sci 2016;99:1584–94.
9. Pohler KG, Peres RF, Green JA, et al. Use of bovine pregnancy associated glycoproteins (bPAGs) to diagnose pregnancy and predict late embryonic mortality in postpartum Nelore beef cows. Theriogenology 2016. https://doi.org/10.1016/j.theriogenology.2016.01.026.
10. Cheung S, Parrella A, Rosenwaks Z, et al. Genetic and epigenetic profiling of the infertile male. PLoS One 2019;14:e0214275.
11. DeJarnette J, Saacke R, Bame J, et al. Accessory sperm: their importance to fertility and embryo quality, and attempts to alter their numbers in artificially inseminated cattle. J Anim Sci 1992;70:484–91.
12. Khatib H, Huang W, Wang X, et al. Single gene and gene interaction effects on fertilization and embryonic survival rates in cattle. J Dairy Sci 2009;92:2238–47.

13. O'Callaghan E, Sánchez J, McDonald M, et al. Sire contribution to fertilization failure and early embryo survival in cattle. J Dairy Sci 2021;104:7262–71.
14. Luckett WP. Ontogeny of the fetal membranes and placenta: their bearing on primate phylogeny. Phylogeny of the primates: a multidisciplinary approach. Springer 1975;157–82.
15. Surani MA, Barton SC, Norris ML. Influence of parental chromosomes on spatial specificity in androgenetic——parthenogenetic chimaeras in the mouse. Nature 1987;326:395–7.
16. Boediono A, Suzuki T, Li L, et al. Offspring born from chimeras reconstructed from parthenogenetic and in vitro fertilized bovine embryos. Mol Reprod Dev: Incorporating Gamete Research 1999;53:159–70.
17. Green JA, Parks TE, Avalle MP, et al. The establishment of an ELISA for the detection of pregnancy-associated glycoproteins (PAGs) in the serum of pregnant cows and heifers. Theriogenology 2005;63:1481–503.
18. Wallace RM, Pohler KG, Smith MF, et al. Placental PAGs: gene origins, expression patterns, and use as markers of pregnancy. Reproduction 2015;149:R115–26.
19. Pohler KG, Geary TW, Johnson CL, et al. Circulating bovine pregnancy associated glycoproteins are associated with late embryonic/fetal survival but not ovulatory follicle size in suckled beef cows. J Anim Sci 2013;91:4158–67.
20. Pohler KG, Green JA, Geary TW, et al. Predicting Embryo Presence and Viability. Adv Anat Embryol Cell Biol 2015;216:253–70.
21. Pohler KG, Peres RFG, Green JA, et al. Use of bovine pregnancy-associated glycoproteins to predict late embryonic mortality in postpartum Nelore beef cows. Theriogenology 2016;85:1652–9.
22. Franco GA, Peres RFG, Martins CFG, et al. Sire contribution to pregnancy loss and pregnancy-associated glycoprotein production in Nelore cows. J Anim Sci 2018;96:632–40.
23. Selvaraju S, Parthipan S, Somashekar L, et al. Occurrence and functional significance of the transcriptome in bovine (Bos taurus) spermatozoa. Sci Rep 2017;7:42392.
24. Franco G, Reese S, Poole R, et al. Sire contribution to pregnancy loss in different periods of embryonic and fetal development of beef cows. Theriogenology 2020; 154:84–91.
25. Elbracht M, Mackay D, Begemann M, et al. Disturbed genomic imprinting and its relevance for human reproduction: causes and clinical consequences. Hum Reprod Update 2020;26:197–213.
26. Johnson M, McConnell J, Blerkom JV. Programmed development in the mouse embryo. Development 1984;83:197–231.
27. Seki Y, Hayashi K, Itoh K, et al. Extensive and orderly reprogramming of genome-wide chromatin modifications associated with specification and early development of germ cells in mice. Developmental biology 2005;278:440–58.
28. Hajkova P, Erhardt S, Lane N, et al. Epigenetic reprogramming in mouse primordial germ cells. Mech Dev 2002;117:15–23.
29. Barton SC, Surani M, Norris M. Role of paternal and maternal genomes in mouse development. Nature 1984;311:374–6.
30. Pereira MHC, Wiltbank MC, Vasconcelos JLM. Expression of estrus improves fertility and decreases pregnancy losses in lactating dairy cows that receive artificial insemination or embryo transfer. J Dairy Sci 2016;99:2237–47.
31. Davoodi S, Cooke RF, Fernandes ACdC, et al. Expression of estrus modifies the gene expression profile in reproductive tissues on day 19 of gestation in beef cows. Theriogenology 2016;85:645–55.

32. Houghton FD, Hawkhead JA, Humpherson PG, et al. Non-invasive amino acid turnover predicts human embryo developmental capacity. Hum Reprod 2002;17:999–1005.
33. Buhi WC. Characterization and biological roles of oviduct-specific, oestrogen-dependent glycoprotein. REPRODUCTION-CAMBRIDGE- 2002;123:355–62.
34. Pohler KG, Geary TW, Atkins JA, et al. Follicular determinants of pregnancy establishment and maintenance. Cell Tissue Res 2012;349:649–64.
35. Perry G, Perry B. Effect of preovulatory concentrations of estradiol and initiation of standing estrus on uterine pH in beef cows. Domest Anim Endocrinol 2008;34:333–8.

# Impact of Sire on Embryo Development and Pregnancy

M. Sofia Ortega, PhD[a],*, Kelsey N. Lockhart, MS[b],
Thomas E. Spencer, PhD[b]

## KEYWORDS

- Sire conception rate • Embryo development • In vitro production • Sire effect
- Arrest • Fertility

## KEY POINTS

- Sires vary in their ability to produce embryos and pregnancies.
- No predictor of sire fertility is available.
- Screening models can be useful to find subfertile sires.

## INTRODUCTION

The use of embryo technologies, particularly in vitro embryo production (IVP) is increasing around the world. Data from the International Embryo Technology Society indicates that just in the past 3 years the use of IVP has increased by about 50% (**Fig. 1**A) compared with in vivo embryo production, with a substantial increase in the United States (**Fig. 1**B). This increase is related to several factors including access to technology, qualified personnel, and an increase in the use of beef embryos in dairy cattle.[1] Nevertheless, the progression of zygotes to the blastocyst stage is still significantly lower in IVP compared with in vivo-derived counterparts (**Fig. 1**C, D).

In vivo, using artificial insemination, about 50% of pregnancy losses occur during the first week of development.[2–4] During this time, a series of coordinated events need to take place for pregnancy to be established. First, the oocyte must enter the oviduct and be fertilized by a capacitated sperm to form a zygote.[5] The zygote will then undergo a series of cleavages while traveling in the oviduct toward the uterine horn as a morula about 5 days after fertilization. The compact morula will start forming a fluid-filled cavity termed a blastocoele, which separates 2 distinct cell populations in the newly formed blastocyst: the inner cell mass, which will later give rise to the embryo proper, and the trophectoderm (TE), which will later give rise to the placenta.[6] The use of embryo transfer can help bypass some of the issues associated with gamete

[a] Department of Animal and Dairy Sciences, University of Wisconsin-Madison, 1675 Observatory Drive; [b] Division of Animal Sciences, University of Missouri, Columbia, MO 65211, USA
* Corresponding author.
*E-mail address:* sofia.ortega@wisc.edu

Vet Clin Food Anim 40 (2024) 131–140
https://doi.org/10.1016/j.cvfa.2023.08.007
0749-0720/24/© 2023 Elsevier Inc. All rights reserved.

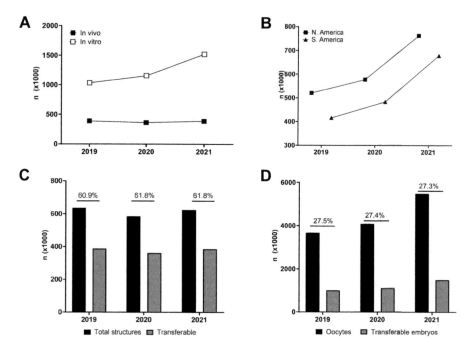

**Fig. 1.** Changes in embryo production from 2019 to 2021. (*A*) Production of embryos in vivo and in vitro from 2019 to 2021. (*B*) IVP in North and South America from 2019 to 2021. (*C*) Production of transferrable embryos in vivo. (*D*) Production of transferrable embryos in vitro from ovum pickup. These data were summarized from the International Embryo Technology Annual Statistics.

and/or embryo failure, including oocyte maturation, gamete transport in the reproductive tract, fertilization ability of the sperm, and embryo competence to progress to the blastocyst stage. In embryo transfer programs, only morphologically "normal" embryos will be transferred into synchronized recipients.[7]

After day 8 of development, the blastocyst will then hatch from the zona pellucida and will progress into an ovoid, and then filamentous shape by day 15 after insemination. The elongating conceptus secretes interferon tau (IFNT) that acts on the endometrium to inhibit the development of the luteolytic mechanism resulting in maternal recognition of pregnancy.[8–10] IFNT also acts in a paracrine manner on the endometrium to induce the expression of IFN-stimulated genes, which are hypothesized to regulate uterine receptivity and conceptus elongation.[11–13] After day 19 in cattle, the TE of the elongating conceptus begins to adhere to the luminal epithelium of the uterus and starts the process of placentation that involves differentiation of trophoblast giant binucleate cells (BNC) and formation of an embryo and extraembryonic membranes.[14,15] Trophoblast BNC are crucial for the formation of placentomes that are vital for fetal and placental growth to term. As they begin to form about day 24, BNC express specific pregnancy-associated glycoproteins (PAGs) that can be detected in maternal circulation and used to diagnose pregnancy and monitor placental function.[16–18] Of note, about 20% of pregnancies are lost between days 8 and 28 of pregnancy.[4] This has been attributed to initial embryo quality, where embryos of higher quality underwent more cleavages by day 7, had more cells that could benefit further development; however, no clear influence of sire has been attributed to conceptus length.[19,20]

Most of the studies so far has been focused on understanding how the maternal environment influences pregnancy establishment, where the most important maternal contribution seems to be the intrinsic quality of the oocyte.[21–23] However, very few studies have investigated the effect of the sire or sire fertility on embryo development and pregnancy establishment. This is likely because of the difficulty of assessing sperm contributions beyond fertilization and current quality controls.

## CONTRIBUTIONS OF THE SIRE TO THE EARLY EMBRYO

The sperm contributes more than just its DNA to the developing embryo. At the time of fertilization, sperm contribute two important pieces to embryo development: the oocyte-activating factor, and the centriole. The oocyte-activating factor signals the calcium oscillation within the oocyte, which is responsible for the resumption of meiosis II and the formation of the female pronucleus. The sperm-specific protein responsible is thought to be phospholipase C-zeta (PLCζ).[24] After the sperm binds to the oocyte, PLCζ activates the phosphoinositide pathway.[25,26] In this pathway, PLCζ cleaves phosphatidyl 4,5-bisphosphate into inositol 1,4,5-triphosphate ($IP_3$) and 1,2-diacylglycerol.[27] Then, $IP_3$ binds the type I $IP_3$ receptor on the endoplasmic reticulum, which stores calcium.[28,29] This binding leads to the release of calcium from the endoplasmic reticulum into the cytoplasm. Calcium then activates calmodulin-dependent protein kinase, which activates the anaphase-promoting complex (APC).[30] After activation, APC tags cyclin B, which regulates maturation promoting factor, to be degraded leading to the completion of metaphase II and entrance into anaphase II to finish meiosis.[31,32]

The sperm also contributes its centriole during fertilization. Centrioles are organelles in the cytoplasm that help form and organize spindle fibers.[33] Two centrioles together form a centrosome, which provides structure to the cell and pulls apart chromatids during mitosis. Oocytes lack functional centrioles but retain a store of centrosomal proteins.[34] At the time of fertilization, activation of the oocyte results in changes in pH and calcium, which will cause centrosome remodeling. The sperm's proximal centriole helps in the recruitment of centrosomal proteins from the oocyte to form the sperm aster, then zygote aster (containing both sperm and female contributions), and the mitotic apparatus.[35,36]

In addition to DNA, centrioles, and proteins, the sperm contain mRNAs and micro-RNAs (miRNAs) that are also delivered to the oocyte during fertilization. It is important to note that although the major wave of embryonic genome activation occurs at the 8 to 16-cell stage in the bovine, some paternal genes are transcribed as early as the 2 to 4-cell stage.[37] Differentially expressed miRNAs have been identified in sperm and 2 to 4-cell embryos from high-fertility and low-fertility sires, indicating sperm RNAs have a direct effect on early embryo development.[37] For example, sperm-borne microRNA-34c is important for zygotic cleavage and acts as a regulator of BCL-2 expression. Inhibiting miRNA-34c caused an increased expression of BCL-2, which has an anti-proliferative function, resulting in reduced zygotic cleavage.[38] Literature also demonstrates that sperm-borne miRNA-216b affects cell proliferation, with lower levels in high-fertility sperm leading to higher levels of its target gene K-RAS in embryos, which promotes cell proliferation.[39] Therefore, the sperm contributes many proteins and RNAs to the embryo, which has the potential to be consequential or favorable toward early embryo development.

In a recent study, embryos were produced in vitro and in vivo using sires classified as high or low fertility. Interestingly, the effect on embryo production in both systems was not consistent with sire classification given that some low-fertility sires produced embryos just as the high-fertility ones.[20] This bears the question of why some low-fertility sires have no issues in fertilization or embryo production but still produce fewer pregnancies. For example, in vitro, fertilization issues might be masked by the IVP system itself, given that the sperm is coincubated directly with the oocytes in a dish with no maternal environment interaction. During this coincubation, capacitating agents such as heparin are added to the medium.[40] In this scenario, sires with low fertility due to gamete transport will benefit from the use of an in vitro system. Nevertheless, there will be sires that will underperform in vitro as well, which can lead to reduced pregnancy rates using embryo transfer technologies.

## CONTRIBUTION OF THE SIRE TO PLACENTA FUNCTION

Another issue could be that embryos from low-fertility sires fail later in pregnancy, such as at the time of placentation. It is well established that in cattle as well as other species several genes of paternal origin are increased (bias) in expression in the placenta or are paternally expressed.[41–43] A proper formation of the placenta is necessary for the establishment of the fetal and maternal interface and subsequently pregnancy maintenance. A study has identified sires classified as low fertility that had increased loss between days 19 and 33 of pregnancy,[20] indicating a connection between sire and pregnancy outcomes during the placentation period. In cattle, PAG are secreted by the binucleated cells of the placenta and are used to monitor placental function. For example, low circulating PAG concentrations by day 30 of pregnancy has been associated with late embryonic mortality in dairy[44] and beef cattle.[45,46] Interestingly, circulating concentrations of PAG seem to be affected by sire, where sires that produced pregnancies with lower circulating concentrations of PAG had increased pregnancy loss.[46] Furthermore, using an in vitro system to grow TE cells (placental epithelial cells) we have been able to find differences in PAG secretion in vitro by sire.[47] In this case, the maternal environment is not present, isolating the sire effects on PAG production. It is not clear at this time if these differences are related to placental mass (more cells) or increased activity of the placental cells and requires further investigation.

## SIRE FERTILITY CLASSIFICATION

Unfortunately, at this time, there is no genomic predictor for sire fertility, which could in part be due to the lack of phenotypes that capture the phenotypes described above, which could be used for association analyses. In dairy sires, fertility classification is done using sire conception rate (SCR). SCR is a phenotypic trait determined by day 70 pregnancy rates, and it is defined as the probability a unit of semen from a given sire will produce a pregnancy compared with the average of all bulls tested.[48] Holstein sires must have at least 300 services in the last 4 years to get an SCR value,[48] which makes SCR an indicator rather than a predictor of male fertility. When calculating SCR, fixed effects of herd, year, state, month, registry status, parity, service number, milk yield, dam, and sire age group, and length of the breeding interval are included.[49] Additionally, random effects of bull stud, mating year, service bull, dam, and inbreeding coefficients of the bull and the potential resulting embryo are included in the model.[49] Other variables such as the quality of heat, the health of the female, and human errors cannot be included in the model,[50] leading to a variation in SCR values and observed conception rates because it is not a direct measure of sire fertility.

For example, if a herd with a 30% conception rate was serviced with a bull of average SCR, the observed conception rate could be between 26% and 34%, which could mean a difference of 80 pregnant cows in a 1000-cow herd.[50] Given that SCR is a phenotype, efforts have been made to dissect the genetic component to create a more accurate measure of sire fertility. Previous studies have identified 14 single nucleotide polymorphisms associated with SCR, all of which are in genes involved in gamete maturation, spermatogenesis, motility, and sperm–oocyte interactions.[51,52] Furthermore, the inclusion of nonadditive effects and functional information show promising statistical methods to predict sire fertility.[37,53–56] However, because SCR is determined by day 70 pregnancy rates, it is hard to determine where pregnancies from low SCR sires fail. For example, low SCR sires that are producing fewer pregnancies than average by day 70 may have an issue in embryo production, elongation, or other pregnancy processes that occur before day 70.[20]

## HOW TO PICK A SIRE FOR IN VITRO OR IN VIVO EMBRYO PRODUCTION AND TRANSFER PROGRAMS?

The major drive to select a sire is its genetic merit. It is likely that if a sire is used in an embryo production system in vitro or in vivo, then that sire has desirable characteristics and/or traits wanted in the herd. Now, the ability of the sire to succeed in producing embryos will depend on all the factors mentioned above. Using SCR alone is not always predictive of embryo development. For example, Lockhart and colleagues[57] used 65 sires with SCR values ranging from −14 to 5.3 and found no relation of SCR with embryo production and a low correlation with cleavage (**Fig. 2**).[57] This indicates that SCR as a trait might be more related to fertilization and early embryo events than the later formation of a blastocyst. However, there were individual sire-driven differences in blastocyst production, which can explain the differences in blastocyst production seen in this and other studies.[19,20,58]

One path moving forward could be to test sires in vitro before using them more extensively in embryo programs. There is evidence that sire differences can be detected in vitro that are maintained in vivo as previously shown by Ortega and colleagues.[20] In another study, sires with high or low ability to produce embryos in vitro were used to produce embryos in vivo. Interestingly, about 50% of the sires maintained the same performance in both systems, particularly those sires with very low performance (**Fig. 3**). This suggests that an in vitro system could be used to prescreen sires for

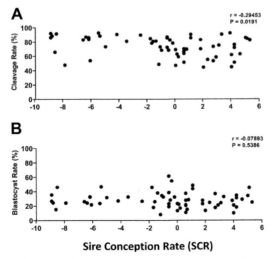

**Fig. 2.** Correlations between SCR value and cleavage and blastocyst production in vitro. (*A*) Correlation of sire SCR value and embryo cleavage in vitro. (*B*) Correlation of SCR value and blastocyst rate in vitro. This was analyzed from data produced by Clark and colleagues.[57]

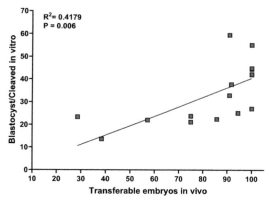

**Fig. 3.** Correlation between the production of transferrable embryos in vitro and vivo using the same sires for both techniques. This graph was reproduced from Clark and colleagues.[57]

noncompensable characteristics that could critically affect embryo development. Similarly, screening of sires for TE growth issues could be done using an in vitro model[47] to identify those that might present a higher risk of pregnancy loss, which will be particularly important for embryo transfer programs. It is important to point out that we are referring to sires with normal or subfertility, the latter being the most challenging to identify given their phenotypic variation explained above. At this moment, a genetic predictor of sire fertility is not yet available; therefore, phenotypic classification will keep playing a big role in sire selection for in vitro and in vivo embryo programs.

## SUMMARY

The use of IVP has increased globally, particularly in the United States. Maternal factors affecting embryo development, such as oocyte quality, have been extensively studied but the influence of the sire on embryo development and pregnancy establishment is less understood. Sperm contributes more than DNA to embryo development, including the oocyte-activating factor and the centriole. The first triggers calcium oscillation necessary for oocyte maturation, whereas the latter helps form spindle fibers and is essential for mitosis. Sperm also delivers mRNAs and microRNAs to the oocyte, which can regulate early embryo development. Recent studies have shown that current sire fertility classification does not consistently correlate with embryo production outcomes. Low-fertility sires may perform well in certain systems, such as IVP, where gamete transport issues are masked but still produce fewer pregnancies. Issues related to fertilization or in vivo embryo production may be masked by the in vitro environment. Furthermore, low-fertility sires may experience failures during later stages of pregnancy, such as placentation, leading to reduced pregnancy rates in embryo transfer programs. When selecting a sire for IVP or embryo transfer programs, genetic merit is a primary consideration. Testing sires in vitro before extensive use in embryo programs may help identify non-compensable characteristics that affect embryo development or sires with a higher risk of pregnancy loss.

## FUNDING

This study was funded by USDA NIFA AFRI Grant 2019-67015-28998, USDA NIFA Grant 2022-67015-36371, and the USDA National Needs Fellowship USDA NIFA Grant 2019-38420-28972.

**CONFLICT OF INTEREST**

The authors declare no conflict of interest.

**REFERENCES**

1. Fuerniss LK, Wesley KR, Bowman SM, et al. Beef embryos in dairy cows: Feedlot performance, mechanistic responses, and carcass characteristics of straight-bred Holstein calves and Angus-sired calves from Holstein, Jersey, or crossbred beef dams. J Anim Sci 2023;skad239. https://doi.org/10.1093/jas/skad239.
2. Cerri RLA, Rutigliano HM, Chebel RC, et al. Period of dominance of the ovulatory follicle influences embryo quality in lactating dairy cows. Reproduction 2009; 137(5):813–23.
3. Cerri RLA, Juchem SO, Chebel RC, et al. Effect of fat source differing in fatty acid profile on metabolic parameters, fertilization, and embryo quality in high-producing dairy cows. J Dairy Sci 2009;92(4):1520–31.
4. Wiltbank MC, Baez GM, Garcia-Guerra A, et al. Pivotal periods for pregnancy loss during the first trimester of gestation in lactating dairy cows. Theriogenology 2016;86(1):239–53.
5. Spencer TE, Hansen TR. Implantation and establishment of pregnancy in ruminants. Adv Anat Embryol Cell Biol 2015;216:105–35.
6. Wei Q, Zhong L, Zhang S, et al. Bovine lineage specification revealed by single-cell gene expression analysis from zygote to blastocyst. Biol Reprod 2017; 97(1):5–17.
7. Hansen PJ. The incompletely fulfilled promise of embryo transfer in cattle—why aren't pregnancy rates greater and what can we do about it? J Anim Sci 2020; 98(11). https://doi.org/10.1093/jas/skaa288.
8. Spencer TE, Burghardt RC, Johnson GA, et al. Conceptus signals for establishment and maintenance of pregnancy. Anim Reprod Sci 2004;82:537–50.
9. Bazer FW, Wu G, Spencer TE, et al. Novel pathways for implantation and establishment and maintenance of pregnancy in mammals. Mol Hum Reprod 2010; 16(3):135–52.
10. Brooks K, Burns G, Spencer TE. Conceptus elongation in ruminants: roles of progesterone, prostaglandin, interferon tau and cortisol. J Anim Sci Biotechnol 2014; 5(1). https://doi.org/10.1186/2049-1891-5-53.
11. Hansen TR, Austin KJ, Perry DJ, et al. Mechanism of action of interferon-tau in the uterus during early pregnancy. J Reprod Fertil Suppl 1999;54:329–39.
12. Spencer TE, Sandra O, Wolf E. Genes involved in conceptus–endometrial interactions in ruminants: insights from reductionism and thoughts on holistic approaches. Reproduction 2008;135(2):165–79.
13. Brooks K, Spencer TE. Biological roles of Interferon Tau (IFNT) and Type I IFN receptors in elongation of the ovine conceptus. Biol Reprod 2015;92(2):47.
14. Davenport KM, Ortega MS, Liu H, et al. Single-nuclei RNA sequencing (snRNA-seq) uncovers trophoblast cell types and lineages in the mature bovine placenta. Proc Natl Acad Sci USA 2023;120(12). e2221526120.
15. Wooding FB. Current topic: the synepitheliochorial placenta of ruminants: binucleate cell fusions and hormone production. Placenta 1992;13(2):101–13.
16. Green JA, Parks TE, Avalle MP, et al. The establishment of an ELISA for the detection of pregnancy-associated glycoproteins (PAGs) in the serum of pregnant cows and heifers. Theriogenology 2005;63(5):1481–503.

17. Pohler KG, Geary TW, Johnson CL, et al. Circulating bovine pregnancy associated glycoproteins are associated with late embryonic/fetal survival but not ovulatory follicle size in suckled beef cows. J Anim Sci 2013;91(9):4158–67.
18. Greenstein JS, Murray RW, Foley RC. Observations on the morphogenesis and histochemistry of the bovine pre-attachment placenta between 16 and 33 days of gestation. Anat Rec 1958;132(3):321–41.
19. O'Callaghan E, Sánchez JM, McDonald M, et al. Sire contribution to fertilization failure and early embryo survival in cattle. J Dairy Sci 2021;104(6):7262–71.
20. Ortega MS, Moraes JGN, Patterson DJ, et al. Influences of sire conception rate on pregnancy establishment in dairy cattle. Biol Reprod 2018;99(6):1244–54.
21. Boni R, Cuomo A, Tosti E. Developmental potential in bovine oocytes is related to cumulus-oocyte complex grade, calcium current activity, and calcium stores. Biol Reprod 2002;66(3):836–42.
22. Rizos D, Ward F, Duffy P, et al. Consequences of bovine oocyte maturation, fertilization or early embryo development in vitro versus in vivo: Implications for blastocyst yield and blastocyst quality. Mol Reprod Dev 2002;61(2):234–48.
23. Rahman MB, Vandaele L, Rijsselaere T, et al. Oocyte quality determines bovine embryo development after fertilisation with hydrogen peroxide-stressed spermatozoa. Reprod Fertil Dev 2012;24(4):608–18.
24. Malcuit C, Kurokawa M, Fissore RA. Calcium oscillations and mammalian egg activation. J Cell Physiol 2006;206(3):565–73.
25. Turner PR, Sheetz MP, Jaffe LA. Fertilization increases the polyphosphoinositide content of sea urchin eggs. Nature 1984;310(5976):414–5.
26. Stith BJ, Espinoza R, Roberts D, et al. Sperm increase inositol 1,4,5-trisphosphate mass in xenopus laevis eggs preinjected with calcium buffers or heparin. Dev Biol 1994;165(1):206–15.
27. Rice A, Parrington J, Jones KT, et al. Mammalian Sperm Contain a Ca2+-Sensitive phospholipase C activity that can generate InsP3 from PIP2 associated with intracellular organelles. Dev Biol 2000;228(1):125–35.
28. Miyazaki S. Inositol 1,4,5-trisphosphate-induced calcium release and guanine nucleotide-binding protein-mediated periodic calcium rises in golden hamster eggs. JCB (J Cell Biol) 1988;106(2):345–53.
29. Berridge MJ. The endoplasmic reticulum: a multifunctional signaling organelle. Cell Calcium 2002;32(5–6):235–49.
30. Yamamoto TM, Iwabuchi M, Ohsumi K, et al. APC/C–Cdc20-mediated degradation of cyclin B participates in CSF arrest in unfertilized Xenopus eggs. Dev Biol 2005;279(2):345–55.
31. Gautier J, Minshull J, Lohka M, et al. Cyclin is a component of maturation-promoting factor from Xenopus. Cell 1990;60(3):487–94.
32. Nixon VL, Levasseur M, McDougall A, et al. Ca2+ oscillations promote APC/C-dependent cyclin B1 degradation during metaphase arrest and completion of meiosis in fertilizing mouse eggs. Curr Biol 2002;12(9):746–50.
33. Azimzadeh J, Marshall WF. Building the centriole. Curr Biol 2010;20(18):R816–25.
34. Sutovsky P, Manandhar G, Schatten G. Biogenesis of the centrosome during mammalian gametogenesis and fertilization. Protoplasma 1999;206(4):249–62.
35. Schatten H, Sun Q. New insights into the role of centrosomes in mammalian fertilization and implications for ART. Reproduction 2011;142(6):793–801.
36. Manandhar G, Schatten H, Sutovsky P. Centrosome reduction during gametogenesis and its significance. Biol Reprod 2005;72(1):2–13.
37. Gross N, Strillacci MG, Peñagaricano F, et al. Characterization and functional roles of paternal RNAs in 2–4 cell bovine embryos. Sci Rep 2019;9(1):20347.

38. Liu WM, Pang RTK, Chiu PCN, et al. Sperm-borne microRNA-34c is required for the first cleavage division in mouse. Proc Natl Acad Sci USA 2012;109(2):490–4.
39. Alves MBR, de Arruda RP, De Bem THC, et al. Sperm-borne miR-216b modulates cell proliferation during early embryo development via K-RAS. Sci Rep 2019; 9(1):1–14.
40. Parrish JJ. Bovine In vitro fertilization: In vitro oocyte maturation and sperm capacitation with heparin. Theriogenology 2014;81(1). https://doi.org/10.1016/j.theriogenology.2013.08.005.
41. Dini P, Kalbfleisch T, Uribe-Salazar JM, et al. Parental bias in expression and interaction of genes in the equine placenta. Proc Natl Acad Sci USA 2021;118(16). e2006474118.
42. Chen Z, Hagen DE, Elsik CG, et al. Characterization of global loss of imprinting in fetal overgrowth syndrome induced by assisted reproduction. Proc Natl Acad Sci USA 2015;112(15):4618–23.
43. Pilvar D, Reiman M, Pilvar A, et al. Parent-of-origin-specific allelic expression in the human placenta is limited to established imprinted loci and it is stably maintained across pregnancy. Clin Epigenet 2019;11(1):94.
44. Pohler KG, Pereira MHC, Lopes FR, et al. Circulating concentrations of bovine pregnancy-associated glycoproteins and late embryonic mortality in lactating dairy herds. J Dairy Sci 2016;99(2):1584–94.
45. Franco G, Reese S, Poole R, et al. Sire contribution to pregnancy loss in different periods of embryonic and fetal development of beef cows. Theriogenology 2020; 154:84–91.
46. Franco GA, Peres RFG, Martins CFG, et al. Sire contribution to pregnancy loss and pregnancy-associated glycoprotein production in Nelore cows. J Anim Sci 2018;96(2):632–40.
47. Ortega MS, Rizo JA, Drum JN, et al. Development of an improved in vitro model of bovine trophectoderm differentiation. Frontiers in Animal Science 2022;3:13. Available at: https://www.frontiersin.org/articles/10.3389/fanim.2022.898808. Accessed April 6, 2023.
48. Norman HD, Hutchison JL, VanRaden PM. Evaluations for service-sire conception rate for heifer and cow inseminations with conventional and sexed semen. J Dairy Sci 2011;94(12):6135–42.
49. Kuhn MT, Hutchison JL. Prediction of dairy bull fertility from field data: Use of multiple services and identification and utilization of factors affecting bull fertility. J Dairy Sci 2008;91(6):2481–92.
50. DeJarnette JM, Amann RP. Understanding estimates of AI sire fertility: From A to Z. In: Proceedings of the 23rd Tech Conference Artific Insem Reprod Natl Assoc Anim Breeders. 2010:13-27.
51. Peñagaricano F, Weigel KA, Khatib H. Genome-wide association study identifies candidate markers for bull fertility in Holstein dairy cattle. Anim Genet 2012;43: 65–71.
52. Han Y, Peñagaricano F. Unravelling the genomic architecture of bull fertility in Holstein cattle. BMC Genet 2016;17(1):143.
53. Abdollahi-Arpanahi R, Morota G, Peñagaricano F. Predicting bull fertility using genomic data and biological information. J Dairy Sci 2017;100(12):9656–66.
54. Nani JP, Rezende FM, Peñagaricano F. Predicting male fertility in dairy cattle using markers with large effect and functional annotation data. BMC Genom 2019; 20(1):258.
55. Schober P, Boer C, Schwarte LA. Correlation Coefficients: Appropriate use and interpretation. Anesth Analg 2018;126(5):1763–8.

56. Kropp J, Carrillo JA, Namous H, et al. Male fertility status is associated with DNA methylation signatures in sperm and transcriptomic profiles of bovine preimplantation embryos. BMC Genom 2017;18(1):280.
57. Clark K. Paternal effects on pre-implantation embryo development in cattle. M.S. University of Missouri–Columbia; 2021. https://doi.org/10.32469/10355/90127.
58. Zoca SM, Walker JA, Kline AC, et al. Relationship of field and in vitro fertility of dairy bulls with sperm parameters, including DAG1 and SERPINA5 proteins. Front Anim Sci 2023;4:1180967.

# Implementing Fixed-Time Artificial Insemination Programs in Beef Herds

Vitor R.G. Mercadante, DVM, MS, PhD[a],*,
Graham Cliff Lamb, MS, PhD[b]

## KEYWORDS

• Estrous synchronization • Artificial insemination • Beef cattle • Pregnancy

## KEY POINTS

• Estrous synchronization and fixed-time artificial insemination (TAI) are impactful reproductive technologies in beef cow-calf production, with the ability to increase pregnancy rates, enhance weaning weights, and improve profitability.

• Adoption of TAI and other reproductive technologies by US beef cow-calf producers has been slow.

• Current TAI protocols yield consistent and satisfactory pregnancy results, but are affected primarily by cow body condition score (BCS) and days postpartum.

• Adoption of breeding programs that include TAI should focus on long-term results with an emphasis on cow and heifer nutritional status, improvement of cattle handling conditions, and selection pressure for fertility.

## INTRODUCTION

The economic success of beef cow-calf operations relies on the ability to produce one live healthy and heavy at weaning calf per cow every year. To achieve this goal, beef cow-calf producers need to overcome several obstacles related to the cow, bull, and the offspring including ovulation and fertilization rates and embryonic, fetal, and postnatal survivals.[1] Over the last five decades several advances in reproductive biotechnologies, such as artificial insemination (AI), estrus-synchronization, and fixed-time AI (TAI), have helped beef producers improve genetic traits of their cattle, tighten the breeding season, and shorten the calving season leading to an increase in overall profitability of cow-calf production systems.[2,3]

Enhanced understanding of the dynamics of the estrous cycle have made possible the development of protocols to manipulate the estrous cycle and control ovulation

[a] School of Animal Sciences, CALS and Large Animal Clinical Sciences, VAMD-CVM at Virginia Tech, 175 West Campus Drive, Blacksburg, VA 24061, USA; [b] Texas A&M Agrilife Research, 600 John Kimbrough Boulevard, College Station, TX 77843, USA
* Corresponding author.
*E-mail address:* mercadante@vt.edu

Vet Clin Food Anim 40 (2024) 141–156
https://doi.org/10.1016/j.cvfa.2023.08.008          vetfood.theclinics.com
0749-0720/24/Published by Elsevier Inc.

with great precision and success by using natural and/or artificially synthesized hormones, such as gonadotropin-releasing hormone (GnRH), prostaglandin $F_{2\alpha}$ (PGF), and progestins. Use of estrus or ovulation synchronization and TAI has facilitated the widespread use of AI and can greatly impact the economic viability of cow-calf systems by increasing total pounds of calf weaned per cow exposed.[3] Implementation of TAI programs by beef producers, however, depends largely on three key factors:

1. Limited frequency of handling cattle
2. Elimination of detection of estrus
3. Satisfactory and consistent pregnancy outcomes

Fixed-time AI is possibly one of the most impactful technologies available to beef cow-calf producers with benefits that go beyond the genetic improvement potential of AI, but also has direct impacts on the cow and their offspring, and allowing for improved labor, nutritional, health, and reproductive management optimization and increased profitability of the operation.

## ADOPTION RATES OF ARTIFICIAL INSEMINATION AND FIXED-TIME ARTIFICIAL INSEMINATION IN THE UNITED STATES

Although the benefits of implementing reproductive management strategies and technologies on beef cow-calf operations are numerous, adoption by beef producers in the United States has been slow. The US Department of Agriculture National Animal Health Monitoring System performed a comprehensive survey of beef cow-calf producers on the health and management of their cattle.[4] This study and survey involved producers from the 24 most prevalent states in beef production, representing more than 70% of beef females and beef operations in the United States.

The survey indicates that overall adoption of reproductive technologies is poor, with only 37.5% of beef operations indicating the use of at least one reproductive technology (**Fig. 1**). The most commonly used reproductive technology is pregnancy diagnosis with 31.6% (using either rectal palpation, ultrasonography, or a blood test [19.3%, 8.8%, and 3.5%, respectively]), followed by semen evaluation of natural service sires performed by a breeding soundness examination with 19.7%. AI is implemented by 11.6% of operations, with only 7.3% of beef cow-calf operations using estrous synchronization to perform AI. In contrast, in the US dairy industry 89.3% of all pregnancies are the result of AI.[5]

The United States has also been surpassed by Brazil, the second largest beef producer in the world, in the use of AI and TAI. Currently, Brazil artificially inseminates

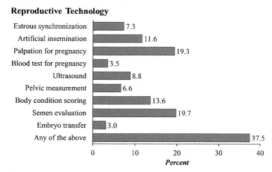

**Fig. 1.** Adoption of reproductive technologies by US beef cow-calf producers. (*Adapted from* NAHMS, 2020.[4])

13.6% of beef females, of which 86% were performed by TAI.[6] With the development of reliable estrous synchronization protocols the use of TAI in beef operations in Brazil has grown 130-fold between 2002 and 2018.[6] In the United States, use of AI in beef operations increased from 7.6% in 2007 to 11.6% in 2017, whereas the use of TAI remained similar (**Fig. 2**).[4,7] The main increase in adoption of estrous synchronization and TAI is seen in medium (between 100 and 199 head) and large (more than 200 head) US beef cow-calf operations with a growth of approximately 10% points from 2007 to 2017 (see **Fig. 2**).[4,7]

Nonetheless, AI and TAI remain mostly underused by US beef cow-calf producers. When queried as to their reluctance to use TAI, more than 53% of beef operations cited labor concerns or complicated estrous synchronization protocols as primary reasons for not implementing this reproductive technology.[4]

## IMPACTS OF ESTROUS SYNCHRONIZATION ON COW-CALF PRODUCTIVITY AND PROFITABILITY

Estrous synchronization and TAI has facilitated the widespread use of AI and can greatly impact the economic viability of cow-calf systems by shortening the breeding season, increasing the proportion of females that are exposed to AI, increasing pregnancy rate earlier in the breeding season, and, consequently, increasing calving rate early in the calving season (**Fig. 3**).[3] This increase in number of calves born earlier in the calving season results in older and heavier calves at weaning, with an increase in weaning weights per cow exposed of 17.5 kg.[3] In that same study, a partial budget analysis revealed an overall increase in net returns of $49.14 per cow exposed for cows exposed to TAI compared with cows exposed to natural breeding only.[3] The increase in net returns is mainly related to a greater calving rate early in the calving season and the ability to reduce the number of bulls needed for natural service following TAI. However, the decrease in costs related to the purchase of bulls assumed that if 50% of the cows became pregnant by TAI, then a producer would be able to reduce the number of bulls in half while maintaining a similar bull to cow ratio for the remainder of cows that failed to become pregnant by TAI. Cows that remain nonpregnant return to estrus in a synchronized manner, with most returning 20 to 23 days post-TAI,[8] and could put added pressure on the bull to breed as many females in a much shorter amount of time.

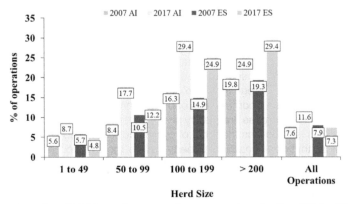

**Fig. 2.** Adoption of artificial insemination and estrus synchronization (ES) by US beef cow-calf producers in 2007 and 2017. (*Adapted from* NAHMS 2008, 2020.[4,5])

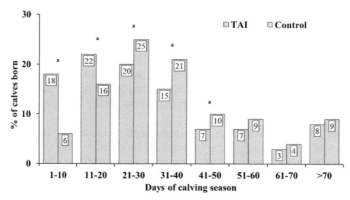

**Fig. 3.** Calving distribution of cows enrolled in a breeding season with (TAI) or without (Control) estrous synchronization. [a]Within 10-day interval treatments differ (*P*<.05). (*Adapted from* Rodgers et al., 2012.[3])

The current recommended bull/cow ratio is 20 to 30 cows in pasture for every one bull.[9,10] However, the average number of beef cows exposed to yearling bulls is reported at 15.2 and for mature bulls at 22.0, regardless of the use of synchronization and TAI.[4] The recommended 1:25 bull/cow ratio may be too conservative and not reaching the bulls full breeding potential, because no changes in pregnancy rates have been reported when nonsynchronized cows were on pasture with bulls in ratios of 1:25, 1:44, or 1:60 bulls per cow.[11] Recently, a retrospective study aimed to determine if the bull/cow ratio affects pregnancy success after estrous synchronization and TAI in beef cattle.[12] Decreasing the bull/cow ratio had a negative correlation with pregnancy rates, but only a small portion of the observed variation (1%–4% for bull to total number of cow ratio, 1%–11% of variation for bull to open cow after TAI ratio) is attributed to the bull/cow ratio. Overall, bull/cow ratios remained similar to 1:30, yet after TAI, the number of open cows that need service was reduced by half. Therefore, a bull/cow ratio of at least 1:50 can be used when implementing estrous synchronization and TAI in combination with natural service using mature bulls that have successfully passed a breeding soundness examination.[12] This decrease in the bull/cow ratio may help alleviate the economic burden of implementing estrous synchronization and TAI, while ensuring an increase in profitability resulting from the greater weaning weights per cow exposed.

## FACTORS AFFECTING PREGNANCY SUCCESS OF FIXED-TIME ARTIFICIAL INSEMINATION

Success of TAI programs is influenced by factors related to the cow or heifer, the sire, and the management system imposed on those females. Postpartum anestrous remains as a large obstacle to increase pregnancy rate of beef females early in the breeding season and TAI protocols that use a combination of progestins, GnRH, and PGF have the ability to induce cyclicity and increase pregnancy rate of anestrous females.[13] However, fertility of anestrous cows is often less than that of cycling cows enrolled in TAI programs.[13,14] Similarly, heifers that have reached puberty before the initiation of the TAI protocol have greater pregnancy rates than heifers that failed to reach puberty.[15]

Nutritional status is closely related to incidence of postpartum anestrous in beef cows and puberty achievement in beef heifers. In beef cows, the two main factors that affect pregnancy success of TAI programs are body condition score (BCS) and days postpartum. A retrospective analysis of several studies[13] indicated that the greatest pregnancy rates to TAI were in mature cows with extended days postpartum (>72 days) and greater than five BCS. Pregnancy rate was similar for cows with days postpartum greater than 72 days and BCS lesser than five, and cows with days postpartum lesser than 72 days and BCS greater than five. However, in both cases pregnancy rate was decreased significantly compared with cows with having greater than 72 days postpartum and greater than five BCS, highlighting the importance of coupling days postpartum and BCS for improved TAI pregnancy success.

In heifers, attainment of puberty depends on age and body weight (BW).[15,16] Heifers are usually developed to a target weight, reaching between 55% and 65% of mature BW. Several studies have compared both targeted BWs, as reviewed by Perry.[15] When heifers are developed to 55% compared with 65% of mature BW, no difference between developmental weights was detected in percentage of heifers reaching puberty at 12 months of age or yearling pregnancy rates after an 80-day breeding season.[17] However, more heifers developed to 65% of mature BW were pregnant during the first 45 days of the breeding season compared with heifers developed to 55% of mature BW.[18] The development target had carry-over effects, where a difference was observed in postpartum interval with heifers developed to 55% of mature BW taking longer to reinitiate postpartum estrous cycles after calving compared with heifers developed to 65% of mature BW.[17] This is of particular importance, because heifers that calve early during their first calving season wean heavier calves for up to six calving seasons and have increased longevity compared with heifers that calve later in their first calving season.[19]

When considering pregnancy success of TAI programs much attention is focused on the female; however, recent studies have demonstrated the impact of sires on pregnancy success through effects on pregnancy loss. Variation on TAI pregnancy rates of sires has been reported from 35% to 55%, for Bos taurus sires that had semen collected, frozen, and successfully passed all prefreezing and postthaw quality tests.[20] For that same study, sires were classified by pregnancy loss as either high with a mean of 7.25% or low with a mean of 3.93%. Paternal genetics play an important role in placenta formation and seem to be critical during later stages of embryonic development.[21,22] Although selection and classification of sires based on TAI pregnancy success is possible, this task will fall largely on the cattle genetic selection and semen industry.

When females exhibit estrus before TAI, fertility and pregnancy is enhanced. Concentration of estradiol increases before estrus behavior and the initiation of standing estrus, and the process of ovulation[23]; it also plays a role in changing the uterine environment to receive the embryo and maintain early embryonic development.[23,24] A meta-analysis with more than 10,000 females and across several estrous synchronization protocols indicated a 27% increase in TAI pregnancy rate when females were detected in estrus before insemination.[25] This study also indicated that BCS and cyclicity status before initiation of the TAI protocol impacted estrus response. Cows with BCS greater than four had increased estrus expression compared with cows with less than four BCS, whereas cows in anestrous had greater estrus expression compared with estrus-cycling cows.[25] Estrus-cycling cows could be at any stage of the estrous cycle at the onset of the TAI synchronization protocol and may not respond and anestrous cows,[26] because of a variable response to the first GnRH injection,[27,28] which impacts synchronization rate and, therefore, expression of estrus.[25]

Cattle temperament has also been shown to impact overall performance, fertility, and pregnancy success of TAI. Adequate handling facilities, personnel training on proper low-stress handling techniques, and increased exposure of animals to handling have been shown to reduce the physiologic response to stress and improve temperament.[29] In addition, cows with adequate temperament have increased pregnancy rates, calving rate, and tend to have increased kilogram of calf weaned per cow exposed.[30] Further-more, Bos taurus beef heifers with adequate temperament had a greater pregnancy rate when enrolled in a TAI protocol (**Fig. 4**).[31] In that study, exposure to handling during the TAI protocol reduced concentration of cortisol of heifers, independent of temperament type, indicating that heifers can be quickly acclimated to frequent handling.[31]

## CURRENT FIXED-TIME ARTIFICIAL INSEMINATION PROTOCOLS FOR BEEF FEMALES

Since the first attempts to synchronize estrus with a single injection of PGF,[32] exten-sive research has been conducted and great advancements in the control of the estrous cycle and synchronization of ovulation of beef females has been achieved.[33] Over the past 50 years, several different protocols for TAI have been developed for beef cows in the United States. This abundance of TAI protocols, however, generated confusion among beef producers, especially because little consistency existed on nomenclature of protocols and products used. In 2002 a group of beef cattle repro-ductive biologists from different universities across the United States created the Beef Reproduction Task Force (BRTF) to combine expertise, improve understanding of the physiologic processes of the estrous cycle, and educate producers and veter-inarians regarding the procedures available to manipulate the estrous cycle and syn-chronization of ovulation.[34] The BRTF also created a short list of recommended estrous synchronization protocols for beef cows and heifers, which was developed based on results of peer-reviewed published research and field data collected by AI and genetics companies. Since then, this protocol list has been reviewed, updated, and published annually on the BRTF Web site (www.beefrepro.org) and all major bovine AI sire catalogs (**Figs. 5** and **6**). Recently, two new protocol sheets have been added by the BRTF and include a list of protocols for AI with detection of estrus and when using natural service, and protocols for the use of sexed semen (**Fig. 7**). When selecting an estrous synchronization and TAI protocol for beef females, using the BRTF protocol sheets is highly recommended.

### Protocols that Combine Estrus Detection and Fixed-Time Artificial Insemination

Typically, these protocols rely on a longer interval between luteolysis (PGF injection and progestin device removal) and TAI, which allow for more females to express estrus before insemination. In such protocols, females that express estrus can be insemi-nated approximately 12 hours from the onset or detection of estrus, or inseminated

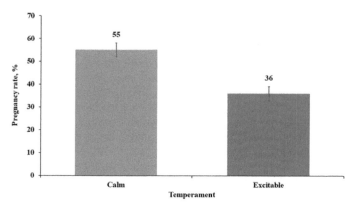

**Fig. 4.** Pregnancy rate of heifers enrolled in TAI according to temperament type. Effect of temperament $P<.05$. (*Adapted from* Dias et al., 2022.[31])

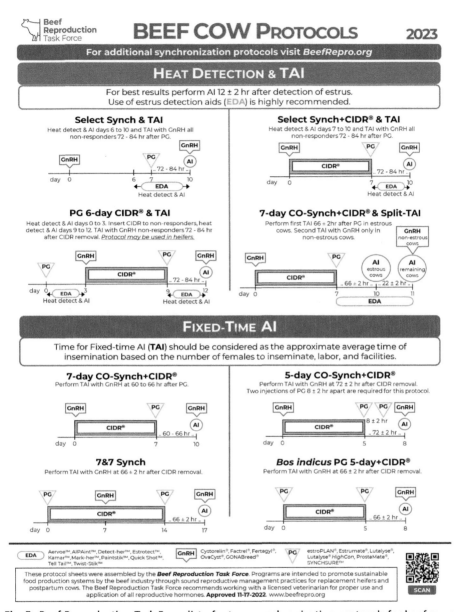

**Fig. 5.** Beef Reproduction Task Force list of estrous synchronization protocols for beef cows.

in two separated TAI events, a strategy that is commonly referred as split-time AI (STAI).[35] Overall pregnancy rates for cows have not been improved when using STAI,[35,36] and results in heifers have been mixed.[36,37] Advantages of estrus detection and TAI, and STAI protocols include the increased proportion of females that are inseminated following estrus expression, and the ability to perform TAI without GnRH injection at the time of AI, which can reduce costs associated with the protocols.[35–37] The main disadvantage of estrus detection and TAI, and STAI protocols is the increased labor associated with estrus detection and extra cattle handling, which

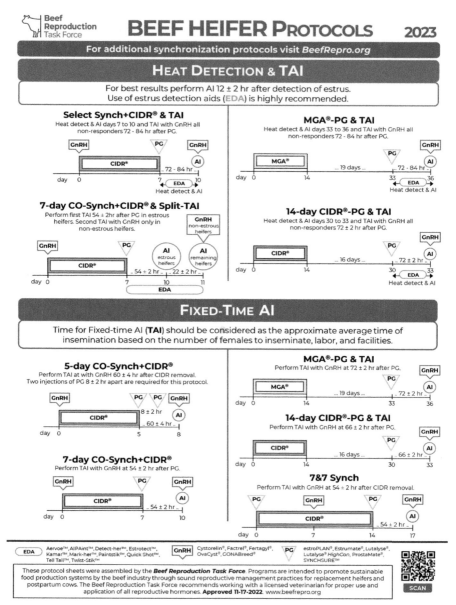

**Fig. 6.** Beef Reproduction Task Force list of estrous synchronization protocols for beef heifers.

may increase the costs associated with the protocol. In addition, when performing estrus detection, the use of estrus detection aids is recommended to improve estrus detection rate.

### Protocols for Fixed-Time Artificial Insemination

The primary advantage of using protocols that rely solely on TAI is the optimization of labor by eliminating estrus detection. For Bos taurus beef cows these protocols tend

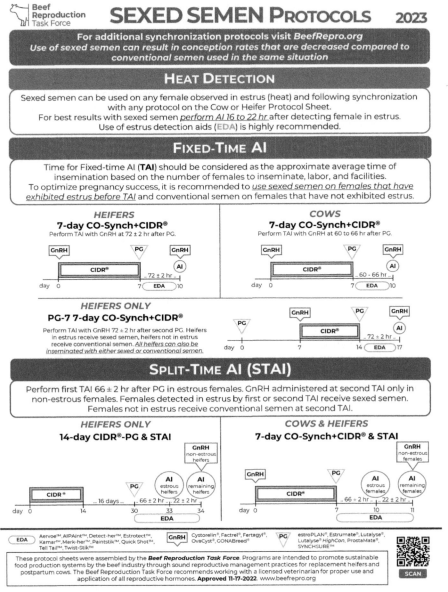

**Fig. 7.** Beef Reproduction Task Force list of estrous synchronization protocols for beef cows and heifers when using sexed-semen.

to be short with approximately 8 to 10 days in duration, including the 7-day CO-Synch + CIDR[38] and the 5-day CO-Synch + CIDR.[39] Comparisons of these two protocols have shown either an advantage in pregnancy rates of the 5-day program[39,40] or similar pregnancy rates between protocols.[13,41]

For beef heifers, TAI protocols can be separated into short- or long-term protocols. Similarly to cows, the two most commonly used short-term protocols are the 7-day CO-Synch + CIDR[42] and the 5-day CO-Synch + CIDR.[39] The two most commonly used long-term protocols are the MGA-PG & TAI and the 14-day CIDR-PG & TAI.[43,44] Reports indicate an increase in synchrony of estrus for long-term TAI protocols in comparison with short-term protocols in beef heifers; however, pregnancy success is similar among protocols.[45]

### Protocols for Presynchronization and Fixed-Time Artificial Insemination

More recently a focus has been set on improving response to the first GnRH injection and consequently ovulation of dominant follicles at the initiation of TAI protocols, improving synchronization of the subsequent follicular waves for cows and heifers.[46] The most successful presynchronization protocols use a combination of PGF injection and prolonged exposure to progesterone to increase ovulation response to first GnRH, improve synchrony, and increase estrus response before TAI in heifers[47] and in cows.[48] The protocol for presynchronization using PGF and the progestin intravaginal insert became commonly known as the 7&7 Synch.[48]

In cows, reports of pregnancy success of the 7&7 Synch in comparison with other TAI protocols have indicated either an improvement[49] or similar results.[50,51] However, in heifers reports of pregnancy success of the 7&7 Synch indicate an improvement in comparison with the 7-day CO-Synch + CIDR protocol.[52]

### Protocols for Use of Sexed Semen

Pregnancy success of TAI protocols using sexed semen is typically between 10% and 20% lower than those of conventional semen,[53] mainly because of the premature onset of sperm capacitation and reduced sperm lifespan in the female reproductive tract.[54] Sexed semen is used with any TAI protocol for cows and heifers; however, insemination with sexed semen is more successful when performed on females that have expressed estrus.[55–57] In addition, a delayed insemination between 16 and 22 hours following onset of estrus is recommended when performing AI based on detection of estrus and with sexed semen.[54–57]

Presynchronization protocols have overall greater estrus response, as previously discussed, and is used strategically with sexed semen insemination of females that express estrus with improved pregnancy success in cows[49] and heifers.[57]

### CONSIDERATIONS FOR IMPLEMENTING FIXED-TIME ARTIFICIAL INSEMINATION IN BEEF COW-CALF OPERATIONS

A common strategy to implement estrous synchronization and TAI in beef cow-calf operations is to start by enrolling only heifers. This allows for producers to familiarize themselves with the TAI procedures, while increasing the proportion of heifers that become pregnant early and calve early, resulting in beneficial long-term effects on weaning weights of the subsequent offspring and their own longevity in the herd.[19] Another strategy is to use synchronization protocols for beef cows in combination with natural service and increase the proportion of cows pregnant early in the breeding season during 1 or 2 years and then enroll cows into a TAI program. This allows for familiarization with synchronization procedures, while helping increase mean calving date and consequently increase days postpartum and improve BCS before the following breeding season, which are essential for TAI pregnancy success.[13] In addition, TAI is implemented in operations that previously relied only on natural service by enrolling heifers into TAI and then forming groups of cows based on their calving dates and enrolling them to TAI, ultimately creating groups of early calving cows that will be exposed to TAI first and groups of late calving cows that are exposed to TAI later in the breeding season. This approach has been previously described in detail by Lamb and

Mercadante[33] and allows for the gradual increase in the proportion of cows that become pregnant early in the breeding season, calve early into the subsequent calving season, and are eligible to enroll into the early TAI group during the following breeding season.

There are several factors that can impact the results of TAI programs, some of which were discussed previously. Pregnancy success varies among different TAI protocols; however, when using protocols that have been established through intense research and tested in thousands of females under different management conditions, the variation in pregnancy success is significantly reduced. Other factors, such as BCS, days postpartum, cyclicity status, and even cattle temperament, become more important for improved TAI pregnancy success.

An important consideration when adopting a TAI breeding program is the need for a long-term commitment with gradual improvements in TAI results. In 2013 we participated in a breeding program that enrolled more than 1500 mature beef cows in eight locations in South Dakota (Lamb and Mercadante, unpublished data). Within location, cows were enrolled using the 7-day CO-Synch + CIDR protocol, were inseminated to the same sires and by the same AI technicians, and pregnancy diagnosis was performed by ultrasonography 35 days post-TAI (**Fig. 8**). Pregnancy rates to TAI varied from 44.4% to 65.8%, with only three locations achieving TAI pregnancy rates greater than 55%. Those three locations had previously used TAI for at least 5 years, whereas the other locations were using TAI for the first time or infrequently and not consistently. In fact, the location with the greatest TAI pregnancy rate (65.8%) had used TAI for the previous 7 years. Prolonged use of TAI results in greater proportion of cows becoming pregnant early in the breeding season, which is intensified over multiple years. The mean days postpartum on the day of AI for the location with the greatest pregnancy success was 87 days with a standard deviation of 5.6 days, whereas for the location with the poorest pregnancy rate the mean days postpartum was 70 days with a standard deviation of 16.9 days. This larger variation in days postpartum affects BCS at TAI, both of which are important to pregnancy success.[13] In addition to the improvements in days postpartum and BCS, long-term exposure to TAI can decrease the stress response of cattle from handling[31] resulting in improved pregnancy results.

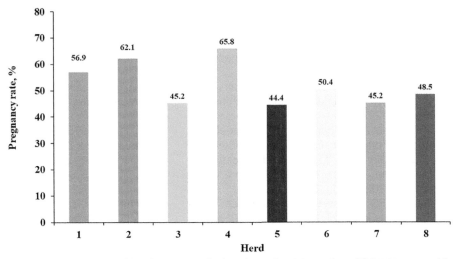

**Fig. 8.** Pregnancy rate of beef cows enrolled in the 7-day CO-synch + CIDR TAI protocol by location (Lamb and Mercadante, unpublished data).

## SUMMARY

Estrous synchronization and TAI remain an important tool to help beef cow-calf producers achieve improved reproductive efficiency, increased weaning weights, and greater net returns. However, adoption of TAI by beef cow-calf producers has been slow when compared with the US dairy industry and other major beef-producing countries, such as Brazil. Advancements in the understanding of the bovine estrous cycle have made possible the development of estrous synchronization programs that have great synchronization rates and deliver consistent pregnancy rates greater than 50%. Although much attention is focused on protocol success, pregnancy success is similar among protocols, whereas other factors, such as BCS and days postpartum, remain of more importance for TAI pregnancy success. Lastly, when adopting TAI programs, a long-term approach must be considered to ensure achievement of greater pregnancy and overall program success.

## CLINICS CARE POINTS

- *Take care of the basics.* A successful fixed-time artificial insemination (TAI) program starts with adequate nutrition, animal health, and a defined breeding season.
- *Walk before you can run.* Start a TAI program with heifers, use estrous synchronization with natural service in cows, and then in the following year consider enrolling all females in TAI.
- *Focus on the long-run.* Define long term reproductive goals, develop a plan, take consistent action and make necessary adjustments in order to achieve the best long-term results.

## DISCLOSURE

The authors have nothing to disclose.

## REFERENCES

1. Inskeep EK, Dailey RA. Embryonic death in cattle. Vet Clin North Am Food Anim Pract 2005;21:437–61.
2. Lamb GC, Dahlen CR, Larson JE, et al. Control of the estrous cycle to improve fertility for fixed-time artificial insemination in beef cattle: a review. J Anim Sci 2010;88:E181–92.
3. Rodgers JC, Bird SL, Larson JE, et al. An economic evaluation of estrous synchronization and timed artificial insemination in suckled beef cows. J Anim Sci 2012;10:1297–308.
4. USDA. Beef 2017, "beef cow-calf management practices in the United States, 2017, report 1. Fort Collins, CO: USDA–APHIS–VS–CEAH–NAHMS; 2020. #.782.0520.
5. USDA. Dairy 2014, "Trends in dairy cattle health and management practices in the United States, 1991-2014". Fort Collins, CO: USDA–APHIS–VS–CEAH–NAHMS; 2021. #711.0821.
6. Baruselli PS, Catussi BLC, de Abreu LA, et al. Challenges to increase the AI and ET markets in Brazil. Anim Reprod 2019;16(3):364–75. https://doi.org/10.21451/1984-3143-AR2019-0050.
7. USDA. Beef 2007-08, Part I: Reference of beef cow-calf management practices in the United States, 2007-08. Fort Collins, CO: USDA-APHIS-VS, CEAH; 2008. #N512-1008.

8. Larson JE, Thielen KN, Funnell BJ, et al. Influence of a controlled internal drug release after fixed-time artificial insemination on pregnancy rates and returns to estrus of nonpregnant cows. J Anim Sci 2009;87(3):914–21.

9. Chenoweth P. 2015. Bull health and breeding soundness. In Bovine Medicine, P.D. Cockcroft (Ed.). doi: 10.1002/9781118948538.ch25.Available at: https://onlinelibrary.wiley.com/action/showCitFormats?doi=10.1002%2F9781118948538.ch25&mobileUi=0.

10. King EH. Management of breeding bull batteries. In: Hopper RM, editor. Bovine reproduction. Ames, IA: Wiley Blackwell; 2015. p. 92–6.

11. Rupp GP, Ball L, Shoop MC, et al. Reproductive efficiency of bulls in natural service: effects of male to female ratio and single- vs multiple-sire breeding groups. J Am Vet Med Assoc 1977;171:639–42.

12. Timlin CL, Dias NW, Hungerford L, et al. A retrospective analysis of bull:cow ratio effects on pregnancy rates of beef cows previously enrolled in fixed-time artificial insemination protocols. Transl Anim Sci 2021;10:1093.

13. Stevenson JS, Hill SL, Bridges GA, et al. Progesterone status, parity, body condition, and days postpartum before estrus or ovulation synchronization in suckled beef cattle influence artificial insemination pregnancy outcomes. J Anim Sci 2015;93:527–40.

14. Stevenson JS, Lamb GC, Johnson SK, et al. Supplemental norgestomet, progesterone, or melengestrol acetate increases pregnancy rates in suckled beef cows after timed inseminations. J Anim Sci 2003;81:571–86.

15. Perry GA. Physiology and endocrinology symposium: harnessing basic knowledge of factors controlling puberty to improve synchronization of estrus and fertility in heifers. J Anim Sci 2012;90(4):1172–82.

16. Garcia MR, Amstalden M, Morrison CD, et al. Age at puberty, total fat and conjugated linoleic acid content of carcass, and circulating metabolic hormones in beef heifers fed a diet high in linoleic acid beginning at four months of age. J Anim Sci 2003;81:261–8.

17. Patterson DJ, Corah LR, Brethour JR, et al. Evaluation of reproductive traits in *Bos taurus* and *Bos indicus* crossbred heifers: effects of postweaning energy manipulation. J Anim Sci 1991;69:2349–61.

18. Patterson DJ, Corah LR, Kiracofe GH, et al. Conception rate in *Bos taurus* and *Bos indicus* crossbred heifers after postweaning energy manipulation and synchronization of estrus with melengestrol acetate and fenprostalene. J Anim Sci 1989;67:1138–47.

19. Cushman RA, Kill LK, Funston RN, et al. Heifer calving date positively influences calf weaning weights through six parturitions. J Anim Sci 2013;91:4486–91.

20. Franco GA, Peres RF, Martins CF, et al. Sire contribution to pregnancy loss and pregnancy-associated glycoprotein production in Nelore cows. J Anim Sci 2018;96(2):632–40.

21. Reese ST, Franco GA, Poole RK, et al. Pregnancy loss in beef cattle: a meta-analysis. Anim Repro Sci 2020;212:106251.

22. Franco G, Reese S, Poole S, et al. Sire contribution to pregnancy loss in different periods of embryonic and fetal development of beef cows. Theriogenology 2020;154:84–91.

23. Perry GA, Perry BL. Effects of standing estrus and supplemental estradiol on changes in uterine pH during a fixed-time artificial insemination protocol. J Anim Sci 2008;86(11):2928–35.

24. Bauersachs S, Ulbrich SE, Gross K, et al. Gene expression profiling of bovine endometrium during the oestrous cycle: detection of molecular pathways involved in functional changes. J Molecular Endo 2005;34:889–908.

25. Richardson BN, Hill SL, Stevenson JS, et al. Expression of estrus before fixed-time AI affects conception rates and factors that impact expression of estrus and the repeatability of expression of estrus in sequential breeding seasons. Anim Repro Sci 2016;166:133–40.

26. Geary TW, Downing ER, Bruemmer JE, et al. Ovarian and estrous response of suckled beef cows to the select synch estrous synchronization protocol. The Professional Animal Scientist 2000;16(1):1–5.

27. Savio JD, Keenan L, Boland MP, et al. Pattern of growth of dominant follicles during the oestrous cycle of heifers. Reproduction 1988;83(2):663–71.

28. Silcox RW, Powell KL, Kiser TE. Ability of dominant follicles (DF) to respond to exogenous GnRH administration is dependent on their stage of development. J Anim Sci 1993;71(Suppl. 1):513.

29. Brandão AP, Cooke RF. Effects of temperament on the reproduction of beef cattle. Animals 2021;11(11):3325.

30. Cooke RF, Bohnert DW, Cappellozza BI, et al. Effects of temperament and acclimation to handling on reproductive performance of *Bos taurus* beef females. J Anim Sci 2012;90:3547–55.

31. Dias ND, Timlin CL, Santilli FV, et al. Effects of temperament on reproductive performance of *Bos taurus* heifers enrolled in the 7-day CO-Synch + controlled internal drug release protocol. Transl Anim Sci 2022;10:1093.

32. Lauderdale JW, Seguin BE, Stellflug JN, et al. Fertility of cattle following PGF2$\alpha$ injection. J Anim Sci 1974;38:964–7.

33. Lamb GC, Mercadante VRG. Synchronization and AI strategies in beef cattle. In: Larson RL, editor. Veterinary Clinics of North America: Food animal Practice. Bovine Theriogenology. Philadelphia, PA: Elsevier; 2016. p. 335–48.

34. Johnson SK, Funston RN, Hall JB, et al. Multi-state Beef Reproduction Task Force provides science-based recommendations for the application of reproductive technologies. J Anim Sci 2011;89(9):2950–4.

35. Thomas JM, Lock SL, Poock SE, et al. Delayed insemination of nonestrous cows improves pregnancy rates when using sex-sorted semen in timed artificial insemination of suckled beef cows. J Anim Sci 2014;92(4):1747–52.

36. Bishop BE, Thomas JM, Abel JM, et al. Split-time artificial insemination in beef cattle: I–Using estrous response to determine the optimal time(s) at which to administer GnRH in beef heifers and postpartum cows. Theriogenology 2016; 86(4):1102–10.

37. Bishop BE, Thomas JM, Abel JM, et al. Split-time artificial insemination in beef cattle: II. Comparing pregnancy rates among nonestrous heifers based on administration of GnRH at AI. Theriogenology 2017;87:229–34.

38. Larson JE, Lamb GC, Stevenson JS, et al. Synchronization of estrus in suckled beef cows for detected estrus and artificial insemination and timed artificial insemination using gonadotropin-releasing hormone, prostaglandin F2$\alpha$, and progesterone. J Anim Sci 2006;84:332–42.

39. Bridges GA, Helser LA, Grum DE, et al. Decreasing the interval between GnRH and PG from 7 to 5 days and lengthening proestrus increases timed-AI pregnancy rates in beef cows. Theriogenology 2008;69:843–51.

40. Whittier WD, Currin JF, Schramm H, et al. Fertility in Angus cross beef cows following 5-day CO-Synch + CIDR or 7-day CO-Synch + CIDR estrus synchronization and timed artificial insemination. Theriogenology 2013;80:963–9.

41. Wilson DJ, Mallory DA, Busch DC, et al. Comparison of short-term progestin-based protocols to synchronize estrus and ovulation in postpartum beef cows. J Anim Sci 2010;88:2045–54.

42. Lamb GC, Larson JE, Geary TW, et al. Synchronization of estrus and artificial insemination in replacement beef heifers using gonadotropin-releasing hormone, prostaglandin F2α, and progesterone. J Anim Sci 2006;84:3000–9.

43. Patterson DJ, Kojima FN, Smith MF. A review of methods to synchronize estrus in replacement heifers and postpartum beef cows. J Anim Sci 2003;81(E. Suppl. 2): E166–77.

44. Leitman NR, Busch DC, Wilson DJ, et al. Comparison of controlled internal drug release insert-based protocols to synchronize estrus in prepubertal and estrous-cycling beef heifers. J Anim Sci 2009;87:3976–82.

45. Patterson DJ, Thomas JM, Locke JWC, et al. Proceedings, Applied Reproductive Strategies in Beef Cattle; August 29-30, 2018; Ruidoso, NM. Available at: https://beefrepro.org/wp-content/uploads/2020/09/PATTERSON-HEIFERS-2018.pdf.

46. Oosthuizen N, Canal LB, Fontes PLP, et al. Prostaglandin F2a 7 d prior to initiation of the 7-d CO-synch + CIDR protocol failed to enhance estrus response and pregnancy rates in beef heifers. J Anim Sci 2018;96:1466–73.

47. Oosthuizen N, Fontes PLP, Porter K, et al. Presynchronization with prostaglandin F2a and prolonged exposure to exogenous progesterone impacts estrus expression and fertility in beef heifers. Theriogenology 2020;146:88–93.

48. Bonacker RC, Stoecklein KS, Locke JW, et al. Treatment with prostaglandin F2α and an intravaginal progesterone insert promotes follicular maturity in advance of gonadotropin-releasing hormone among postpartum beef cows. Theriogenology 2020;157:350–9.

49. Andersen CM, Bonacker RC, Smith EG, et al. Evaluation of the 7 & 7 Synch and 7-day CO-Synch + CIDR treatment regimens for control of the estrous cycle among beef cows prior to fixed-time artificial insemination with conventional or sex-sorted semen. Anim Repro Sci 2021;235:106892.

50. Pancini S, Dias NW, Currin J, et al. Estrus response and pregnancy rates of beef cows enrolled in two fixed-time artificial insemination protocols, with or without pre-synchronization. J Anim Sci 2022;100(Supplement_3):255.

51. Ketchum JN, Quail LK, Epperson KM, et al. Evaluation of two beef cow fixed-time AI protocols that utilize pre-synchronization. J Anim Sci 2022;100(Supplement_3): 139–40.

52. Mercadante VR, Lamb GC, Oosthuizen N, et al. Estrus response and pregnancy rates of beef replacement heifers enrolled in two fixed-time artificial insemination protocols, with or without pre-synchronization. J Anim Sci 2021;99(Supplement_3): 125–6.

53. Oosthuizen N, Porter K, Burato S, et al. Effects of pre-synchronization with prostaglandin F2_ and a progestin, and delayed insemination on pregnancy rates with sexed semen in replacement beef heifers. Front Anim Sci 2022;3: 870978.

54. Bombardelli GD, Soares HF, Chebel RC. Time of insemination relative to reaching activity threshold is associated with pregnancy risk when using sex-sorted semen for lactating Jersey cows. Theriogenology 2016;85:533–9.

55. Thomas JM, Locke JW, Bonacker RC, et al. Evaluation of SexedULTRA 4M™ sex sorted semen in timed artificial insemination programs for mature beef cows. Theriogenology 2019;123:100–7.

56. Perry GA, Walker JA, Rich JJ, et al. Influence of Sexcel™ (gender ablation technology) gender-ablated semen in fixed-time artificial insemination of beef cows and heifers. Theriogenology 2020;146:140–4.

57. Oosthuizen N, Fontes PL, Oliveira Filho RV, et al. Pre-synchronization of ovulation timing and delayed fixed-time artificial insemination increases pregnancy rates when sex-sorted semen is used for insemination of heifers. Anim Repro Sci 2021;226:106699.

# Frozen Bovine Semen Storage, Semen Handling, and Site of Deposition

Joseph C. Dalton, PhD

## KEYWORDS

- Bovine • Semen • Semen handling • Semen deposition

## KEY POINTS

- Artificial insemination (AI) is an effective strategy to improve the genetics and reproductive performance of a herd.
- The liquid nitrogen semen storage tank must be managed properly to realize the maximal potential fertility within straws of frozen semen.
- When retrieving a straw, the cane (and canister) of frozen semen should be held below the frost-line in the neck of the tank.
- Deposit semen in the uterus within approximately 5 minutes (sexed semen) or 10 to 15 minutes (conventional semen) after thawing.
- Manipulation of the reproductive tract must continue until the AI gun tip is past the cervix and semen can be depositedinto the uterine body.

## INTRODUCTION

Artificial insemination (AI) is an effective strategy to distribute semen from genetically elite sires and improve the genetics and reproductive performance of a herd. Commercial AI stud and custom semen collection businesses, through stringent collection, processing, and quality control, provide a highly fertile semen product to their customers. Once transferred to the producer's liquid nitrogen semen storage tank, the maintenance of sire fertility is the responsibility of the owner, employees, and AI technicians.

## SEMEN STORAGE

The liquid nitrogen semen storage tank must be managed properly to realize the maximal potential fertility within straws of frozen semen. The semen storage tank is actually a "tank within a tank," with insulation under vacuum between the inner and

Animal, Veterinary, and Food Sciences Department, University of Idaho, 1904 East Chicago Street, Suite AB, Caldwell, ID 83605, USA
*E-mail address:* jdalton@uidaho.edu

Vet Clin Food Anim 40 (2024) 157–165
https://doi.org/10.1016/j.cvfa.2023.08.009
0749-0720/24/© 2023 Elsevier Inc. All rights reserved.

outer tanks. Liquid nitrogen semen storage tanks should be housed in a clean and dry area. The tank should be securely fastened during transportation to avoid tipping over and damaging the tank, both of which usually results in the loss of liquid nitrogen. A detailed inventory of semen should be easily accessible, regardless of whether the tank is housed in an office or transported to a location closer to the cows to be serviced, so that straws may be removed from the tank quickly to avoid exposure of semen to ambient temperature.

When removing a semen straw from a storage tank, it is imperative that the technician keep the canister, cane, and unused semen straws as low as possible in the neck of the tank. A best management practice is to keep all straws below the frost-line in the neck of the tank. Although the temperature of liquid nitrogen is −196°C, there is a temperature gradient in the neck of the tank.[1] For example, a tank with a neck tube that measures 15.24 cm long may have a temperature of −75°C in the middle of the neck (7.62 cm below the top), while the temperature at 2.54 cm below the top may be −15°C.[1]

A recent study provides evidence the temperature in the neck of a semen storage tank, especially in the area below the frost-line, exhibits wide variation and is influenced by liquid nitrogen level.[2] Berndtson and colleagues[3] repeatedly raised and lowered semen straws in a storage tank and reported the tank's liquid nitrogen level had a dramatic effect on straw temperature. When a tank was full of liquid nitrogen, elevation of a cane (containing a goblet with 5 semen straws) into the neck of the tank for 1 minute resulted in a straw temperature increase of 16°C from −196°C to −180°C.[3] Even after 5 repetitions, the straw temperature reached −196°C within 1 minute, illustrating the effect of a fully charged liquid nitrogen tank.

When the liquid nitrogen level in the tank was low (14 cm), Berndtson and colleagues[3] reported the temperature of straws increased 73°C, from −196°C to −123°C during the first minute, and straw temperatures cooled only 30°C to 40°C 2 minutes after returning to the tank. Consequently, greater temperatures were reached during the second, third, fourth, and fifth repetitions. Berndtson and colleagues[3] reported greater than 10 minutes were required for the straw temperature to reach −196°C upon return after the fifth repetition. Consequently, another best management practice is to monitor the tank's liquid nitrogen level regularly and never let the level of liquid nitrogen go below 25.4 cm.

The ice pattern within bovine semen extender may change considerably (termed recrystallization) as it is warmed.[4] Larger, extracellular ice crystals are associated with damage to sperm cell membranes and organelles,[5] and previous reports have shown that sperm injury (as judged by sperm motility) occurs at temperatures as low as −79°C.[6–8]

When a 0.5-mL straw of semen was raised into the neck of a tank using tweezers, the time interval for the temperature to change from −196°C to −100°C was 10 seconds.[1] Therefore, to avoid recrystallization injury to sperm in straws (not removed from the same goblet or canister), the recommendation is to hold a cane (or canister containing canes) of frozen semen a maximum of 8 seconds in the neck of a tank (below the frost-line) when retrieving straws.[3,5,9]

Other straws on the cane may be exposed to detrimental high temperatures depending on how long it takes to remove a straw.[10] Carelessly working above the frost-line will likely result in sperm damage even when applying the 8-second rule, as straw temperatures will rapidly enter the danger zone.[3,5,9] Injury to sperm cannot be corrected by returning semen to liquid nitrogen[3,9]; therefore, improper straw retrieval leads to additive sperm damage in straws not removed.[3,5,10]

## SEMEN HANDLING

While maintaining the canister and canes below the frost-line, the desired semen straw should be removed with tweezers. The use of fingers, instead of tweezers, is not recommended as this strategy tends to result in the canister and canes being raised above the frost-line. Place the straw immediately in warm water (35°C–37°C) for 45 seconds (in the absence of specific AI stud recommendations). Warm the AI gun either by friction (stroking vigorously with a clean paper towel), placement in a temperature-controlled gun warmer, or by placing it close to your body before loading the straw. Remove the straw from the thaw bath, wipe dry with a clean paper towel, and insert the cotton plug end into the AI gun. Next, cut the straw about 7 mm below the crimped end and place a sheath over the loaded AI gun. To provide thermal protection, place the loaded AI gun in a temperature-controlled gun warmer or wrap it in a clean paper towel and place it close to your body. For a detailed, step-by-step review of semen handling, please see Dalton.[11]

Currently, the majority of bovine semen is processed in either 0.25- or 0.5-mL French straws. The shape and size of these straws facilitate uniform freezing and thawing, leading to improved post-thaw live sperm recovery compared with glass ampules. Unfortunately, the 0.25-mL straw, with a larger surface-to-volume ratio than 0.5-mL straws, is more vulnerable to temperature fluctuations. Consequently, inappropriate semen handling may negatively affect fertility of 0.25-mL straws to a greater degree than mishandling 0.5-mL straws.[3]

A German study classified AI technicians as "good" or "poor" based on nonreturn rates before an AI field trial.[12] (Nonreturn rate, historically used by the dairy industry, is an indirect measure of fertility, specifically defined by Rycroft[13] as the percentage of cows that are not rebred within a specified period of time after an insemination, typically 60–90 days.) Nonreturn rates of "good" technicians were similar for the 0.25- and 0.5-mL straws; however, "poor" technicians achieved a greater nonreturn rate for 0.5-mL than for 0.25-mL straws.[12] Kuperferschmied[12] argued these results provided evidence that 0.25-mL straws were more sensitive to improper semen handling by "poor" technicians. In a meta-analysis, however, fertility following AI with conventional semen in 0.25-mL straws (13 studies, >770,000 inseminations) revealed an advantage of less than 1% for the 0.25-mL package compared with semen in 0.5-mL straws.[14]

Timed AI (TAI) breeding protocols in beef and dairy cattle have become common practice. To facilitate AI of numerous animals in a timely manner on the same day, AI technicians routinely thaw multiple straws of semen simultaneously.

Oliveira and colleagues[15] investigated the effect of the sequence of insemination after simultaneous thawing of 10 straws of conventional semen on pregnancy per AI (P/AI) to TAI in suckled multiparous Nelore cows. Semen from 1 of 3 bulls resulted in decreased fertility for straws 7, 8, 9, and 10; however, fertility of the other 2 bulls was not different across all 10 straws.[15] The results of extensive laboratory analyses of the semen failed to explain the observed decrease in fertility. Oliveira and colleagues[15] concluded that sequence of insemination after simultaneous thawing of 10 straws of conventional semen differentially affected P/AI following TAI, depending on sire.

In a field trial with lactating Holstein dairy cattle, Dalton and colleagues[16] investigated (1) the effect of simultaneous thawing of multiple 0.5-mL straws of conventional semen and sequence of insemination (first, second, third, or fourth) on P/AI, (2) whether P/AI achieved following AI by herdsman-inseminators and professional technicians differed, and (3) the effect of elapsed time from initiation of thawing straws of conventional semen to seminal deposition on P/AI. The average P/AI differed between herdsman-inseminators and professional technicians (27% vs 45%); however, simultaneous thawing and sequence of insemination (first through fourth) and elapsed time from initial thaw to completion of fourth AI had no effect on P/AI within the inseminator group.[16] The elapsed time from initial thaw to completion of fourth AI was shorter for professional technicians than for herdsman-inseminators (7.6 vs 10.9 minutes).[16] Nevertheless, the lower P/AI observed following AI by herdsman-inseminators was not likely due to an extended time factor. Kaproth and colleagues[17] reported that when 0.5-mL conventional semen straws were held at a constant temperature (35°C) after thawing, no difference in mean progressive sperm motility at 5 and 20 minutes post-thaw was observed. In contrast, a decrease in mean progressive sperm motility from 5 to 20 minutes post-thaw was reported when 0.5-mL conventional semen straws were thawed at 35°C but held at 22°C.[17] It is possible that failure to maintain straws at a constant temperature during AI gun assembly and transport to the cow is one of the contributing factors to the decreased fertility seen following AI by herdsman-inseminators.[16]

The 0.25-mL straw was used during the development of sexed semen because of the advantage in post-thaw survival of low sperm dosages due to uniform freezing and thawing rates.[18] Consequently, sexed semen is processed in 0.25-mL straws throughout the world. The large surface-to-volume ratio of the 0.25-mL straw, coupled with the highly processed nature of sexed semen, must be recognized as a contributing factor to the vulnerability of sexed semen to inappropriate handling. When 0.25-mL sexed semen straws were thawed at 35°C and held at either 42°C or 4°C (simulating heat shock and cold shock conditions, respectively), decreased progressive sperm motility at 10 and 15 minutes post-thaw was reported.[19] Similar to conventional semen,[17] no difference in progressive sperm motility was observed when sexed semen was held at a constant temperature (37°C).[19] Taken together, a reasonable strategy to maintain progressive sperm motility (and ultimately, fertility) is to provide appropriate thermal protection to sexed semen straws and deposit semen in the uterus within approximately 5 minutes after thawing.

A recommendation as to the number of straws that may be thawed simultaneously is not appropriate, as time from initial thaw to semen deposition remains an important factor. Therefore, fertility is likely to be maximized when personnel (1) accurately identify cows and heifers in estrus, (2) administer appropriate treatments to synchronize ovulation for TAI, (3) follow the AI stud's recommendations for thawing semen, (4) prevent direct straw-to-straw contact during thawing to avoid decreased post-thaw sperm viability as a result of straws freezing together,[20] (5) use appropriate hygienic procedures, (6) maintain thermal protection of straws during AI gun assembly and transport to the cow, and (7) deposit semen in the uterus within approximately 5 minutes (sexed semen) or 10 to 15 minutes (conventional semen) after initial thawing.

## SITE OF SEMEN DEPOSITION

The objective of insemination (AI and natural service) is to ensure an adequate reservoir of competent, capacitated, motile sperm in the oviductal isthmus at the time of ovulation to facilitate fertilization and pregnancy.[21]

Before discussing the site of semen deposition when performing AI, it is important to briefly discuss the timing of AI. Dalton and colleagues[22] investigated the effect of insemination time on fertilization status and embryo quality in nonlactating, single-ovulating Holstein cows. All cows were continuously monitored by HeatWatch (as described by Walker and colleagues[23]) and received AI with one 0.5-mL straw ($\sim$25 $\times$ 10$^6$ sperm) of conventional semen from 1 of 3 bulls at 0, 12, or 24 hours after the onset of standing estrus, or natural service (hand-mating) at 0 hour.[22] Due to logistics of monitoring the computer software and animal retrieval from pasture, actual insemination times were approximately 2 hours for 0-hour AI and 0-hour natural service and 12 and 24 hours for the remaining treatments.[22] Embryos and ova were recovered 6 to 7 days after insemination using standard nonsurgical uterine-flushing techniques.

The fertilization rate was 98% for the 0-hour natural service treatment, and greater than 70% of embryos were of excellent or good quality.[22] In contrast, fertilization rates were 66% (0-hour AI), 74% (12-hour AI), and 82% (24-hour AI); however, embryo quality declined with increasing intervals after the onset of standing estrus, from high-quality embryos (0-hour AI) to low-quality embryos (24-hour AI).[22] The high proportion of excellent and good embryos resulting from 0-hour AI would be expected to establish pregnancies. As a point of reference, fertilization rates following AI range from 55% to 88% in high-producing dairy cows[24] to greater than 90% in heifers, beef, and moderate-yielding dairy cattle.[25]

The reason the 0-hour natural service treatment was superior in fertilization rate is unknown; however, Dalton and colleagues[22] speculated it may be related to (1) volume, and or components of seminal plasma, in concert with the number of sperm in the ejaculate, (2) potential of recently ejaculated sperm to remain functional longer than frozen sperm, and (3) sperm selection by the cervix and mucus, leading to an increased population of morphologically normal and, perhaps, more competent sperm competing for fertilization.

Embryo quality at the 24-hour AI may be impaired due to an aging ovum at fertilization.[22] In this scenario, 24-hour AI would result in sperm reaching the site of fertilization at 30+ hours after the onset of standing estrus, accounting for the time required for sustained sperm transport (6–12 hours).[26–28] Consequently, fertilization of an aging ovum would occur, likely leading to lower embryo quality. In contrast, the improved embryo quality associated with 0-hour AI suggests that further selection pressure favoring competent sperm may occur as a consequence of increased duration of sperm residence in the female reproductive tract, thus optimizing embryo quality at early insemination.[22] Nevertheless, the low fertilization rate associated with 0-hour AI is likely related to inadequate sperm longevity.

AI at approximately 12 hours after the onset of standing estrus may provide a compromise between the potentially lower fertilization rate of 0-hour AI and the lowered embryo quality of 24-hour AI. From these data, fertility would be expected to be optimized following the 12-hour AI. This agrees with the study by Dransfield and colleagues,[29] in which the optimal time of AI for lactating dairy cows identified in estrus by HeatWatch (DDx Inc., Boulder, CO, USA) was 4 to 16 hours after the onset of estrus. This also agrees with the results of Maatje and colleagues[30] who described an optimal time of insemination between 6 and 17 hours after an increase in activity as monitored by pedometry.

Many studies have compared conventional semen deposition near the greater curvature of the uterine horns with deposition into the uterine body (for a review, see the study by Diskin[21]). Senger and colleagues,[31] López-Gatius,[32] and Pursley[33] reported increased P/AI when conventional semen was deposited in the uterine horns rather than the uterine body. Nevertheless, Hawk and Tanabe,[34] Williams and colleagues,[35] and McKenna et al[36] found no difference in fertility when comparing uterine body and uterine horn inseminations. Furthermore, Diskin and colleagues[37] reported an inseminator and site of conventional semen deposition effect (interaction), with evidence of an increase, decrease, or no effect of uterine horn deposition on P/AI for individual inseminators.

Deposition in the uterine horns might logically be thought of as advantageous, especially relative to reduction of sperm loss by retrograde flow, therefore, potentially enhancing the sperm reservoir in the oviductal isthmus. This does not appear to be true, however, as Gallagher and Senger[38] did not observe a reduction in retrograde sperm loss after semen deposition in the uterine horns compared to the uterine body.

Meirelles and colleagues,[39] using conventional semen in Nelore cows, reported increased fertility following deep intrauterine AI in the horn ipsilateral to the dominant follicle, as compared with seminal deposition in the uterine body. In contrast, Carvalho and colleagues[40] reported deposition of conventional semen in the uterine horns failed to improve fertilization rates in superovulated Holstein cows. Lastly, there is no evidence that sexed semen deposition into the uterine horns enhances fertility as compared with deposition into the uterine body.[41,42]

An explanation for the positive effect of uterine horn inseminations in a few of the aforementioned studies may be related to the minimization or elimination of cervical semen deposition. Cervical insemination errors account for approximately 20% of attempted uterine body depositions.[43] Macpherson[44] reported that cervical insemination resulted in a 10% decrease in fertility when compared with deposition of semen in the uterine body. Gallagher and Senger[38] reported similar retrograde sperm loss among uterine horn and uterine body deposition; however, they observed increased retrograde sperm loss following mid-cervical deposition. Furthermore, in a review by Diskin,[21] the largest improvements in P/AI following uterine horn deposition were achieved by inseminators with the lowest P/AI following uterine body insemination (likely because they were making cervical deposition errors when attempting uterine body deposition).

All AI personnel must develop sufficient skill to recognize when the tip of the AI gun remains in the cervix. To maximize fertility, manipulation of the reproductive tract must be continued until the tip of the AI gun is past the cervix and deposition into the uterus can be accomplished. The importance of retraining, however, cannot be minimized, especially when great variation in fertility levels obtained by technicians, as compared with others, is evident.

King and Macpherson[45] described a situation where the initial training of technicians was deficient and little effort had been made to improve their skill. Excised reproductive tracts and AI guns with dye-filled straws were used, and King and Macpherson[45] reported approximately 25% accuracy of technicians in placing the dye in the uterine body. After initial retraining, the accuracy of technicians increased to 67%.[45] Retraining was continued every 3 months until 80% to 85% accuracy of dye placement in the uterine body was achieved.[45] Not surprisingly, a strong relationship between technician accuracy with dye placement and subsequent fertility has been reported.[45-47] These results provide evidence that retraining can increase the skill level of technicians. Senger[48] stated programs for evaluation of AI skill and retraining using excised tracts should be conducted annually.

## SUMMARY

Appropriate semen storage and handling are critical to the success of an AI program, through maintenance of fertility within straws of frozen semen. Fertility will be maximized when insemination occurs at a time and location that allows for adequate numbers of sperm to be present in the oviducts at the time of ovulation.

## DISCLOSURE

The author states no conflict of interest. Select Sires, Inc. (Plain City, OH, USA), National Association of Animal Breeders (Columbia, MO, USA), and the Virginia Agricultural Council (Richmond, VA, USA) funded the research investigating time of insemination on fertilization rate and embryo quality in non-lactating cows. Select Sires, Inc. funded the research investigating multiple straw thawing and sequential insemination number on fertility in lactating cows, and the effect of liquid nitrogen level on temperature in a semen storage tank.

## REFERENCES

1. Saacke RG, Lineweaver JA, Aalseth EP. Procedures for handling frozen semen. In: Proc. 12th Conf. on AI in Beef Cattle. Columbia, MO: AI in Beef Cattle; 1978. p. 46–61.
2. Ahmadzadeh A, Hale A, Shaffi B, et al. The effect of liquid nitrogen level on the temperature in a semen storage tank. J Dairy and Vet Sci 2022;15(2):555906.
3. Berndtson WE, Pickett BW, Rugg CD. Procedures for field handling of bovine semen in plastic straws. In: Proc. Nat'l. Assoc. Anim. Breeders 6th Tech. Conf. Columbia, MO: Artif. Insem. and Reprod.; 1976. p. 51–60.
4. Rapatz GL. What happens when semen is frozen. In: Proc. Nat'l Assoc. Anim. Breeders 1st Tech. Conf. Columbia, MO: Artif. Insem. and Reprod; 1966. p. 54–63.
5. Stroud B. Consequences of mishandling frozen semen and embryos. In: Proc. Appl. Reprod. Des Moines, IA: Strat. in Beef Cattle; 2016. p. 119–30.
6. Etgen WM, Ludwick JM, Rickard HE, et al. Use of mechanical refrigeration in preservation of bull semen. J Dairy Sci 1957;40:774–8.
7. Bean BH, Pickett BW, Martig RC. Influence of freezing methods, extenders and storage temperatures on motility and pH of frozen bovine semen. J Dairy Sci 1963;46:145–9.
8. DeJarnette JM. Factors affecting the quality of frozen semen after thawing. In: Proc. Soc. for Therio. Nashville, TN: Ann. Conf.; 1999. p. 267–79.
9. Saacke RG. Factors affecting spermatozoan viability from collection to use. In: Proc. Nat'l Assoc. Anim. Breeders 7th Tech. Conf. Columbia, MO: Artif. Insem. and Reprod; 1978. p. 3–9.
10. Saacke RG. Concepts in semen packaging and use. In: Proc. 8th Conference. Columbia, MO: AI in Beef Cattle; 1974. p. 11–9.
11. Dalton JC. Breeding your own cows. In: Dairy Cattle Fertility. Fort Atkinson, WI: WD Hoard and Sons, Co.; 2020. p. 73–5.
12. Kupferschmied H. Untersuchungen uber die umstellung von mittleren auf feine pailletten in der rinderbeasamung. Zuchthygiene 1972;7:67–71.
13. Rycroft H. Factors influencing non-return data. In: Proc. Nat'l. Assoc. Anim. Breeders 14th Tech. Conf. Columbia, MO: Artif. Insem. and Reprod.; 1992. p. 43–6.
14. Stevenson JS, Higgins JJ, Jung Y. Pregnancy outcome after insemination of frozen-thawed bovine semen packaged in two straw sizes: A meta-analysis. J Dairy Sci 2009;92:4432–8.
15. Oliveira LZ, Arruda RP, de Andrade AFC, et al. Effect of sequence of insemination after simultaneous thawing of multiple semen straws on conception rate to timed AI in suckled multiparous Nelore cows. Theriogenology 2012;78:1800–13.
16. Dalton JC, Ahmadzadeh A, Shafii B, et al. Effect of thawing multiple 0.5-mL semen straws and sequential insemination number on conception rates in dairy cattle. J Dairy Sci 2004;87:972–5.
17. Kaproth MT, Parks JE, Grambo GC, et al. Effect of preparing and loading multiple insemination guns on conception rate in two large commercial dairy herds. Theriogenology 2002;57:909–21.

18. Kroetsch TG. Experiences with mini-straws. In: Proc. Nat'l Assoc. Anim. Breeders 14th Tech. Conf. Columbia, MO: Artif. Insemin. and Reprod; 1992. p. 64–7.

19. ABS Global. Achieving maximum semen fertility with ABS Sexation. 2009. Available at: http://www.abstechservices.com/?pages=library. Accessed March 31, 2023.

20. Brown DW, Senger PL, Becker WC. Effect of group thawing on post-thaw viability of bovine spermatozoa packaged in .5-milliliter French straws. J Anim Sci 1991; 69:2303–9.

21. Diskin MG. Review: Semen handling, time of insemination and insemination technique in cattle. Animal 2018;12(S1):75–84.

22. Dalton JC, Nadir S, Bame JH, et al. Effect of time of insemination on number of accessory sperm, fertilization rate, and embryo quality in nonlactating dairy cattle. J Dairy Sci 2001;84:2413–8.

23. Walker WL, Nebel RL, McGilliard ML. Time of ovulation relative to mounting activity in dairy cattle. J Dairy Sci 1996;79:1555–61.

24. Santos JEP, Thatcher WW, Chebel RC, et al. The effect of embryonic death rates in cattle on the efficacy of estrus synchronization programs. Anim Reprod Sci 2004;82-83:513–35.

25. Diskin MG, Waters SM, Parr MH, et al. Pregnancy losses in cattle: Potential for improvement. Reprod Fert Develop 2016;28:83–93.

26. Hawk HW. Transport and fate of spermatozoa after insemination of cattle. J Dairy Sci 1987;70:1487–503.

27. Hunter RHF, Wilmut I. The rate of functional sperm transport into the oviducts of mated cows. Anim Reprod Sci 1983;5:167–73.

28. Wilmut I, Hunter RHF. Sperm transport into the oviducts of heifers mated early in oestrus. Reprod Nutr Dev 1984;24:461–5.

29. Dransfield MBG, Nebel RL, Pearson RE, et al. Timing of insemination for dairy cows identified in estrus by a radiotelemetric estrus detection system. J Dairy Sci 1998;81:1874–82.

30. Maatje K, Loeffler SH, Engel B. Predicting optimal time of insemination in cows that show visual signs of estrus by estimating onset of estrus with pedometers. J Dairy Sci 1997;80:1098–105.

31. Senger PL, Becker WC, Davidge ST, et al. Influence of cornual insemination on conception in dairy cattle. J Anim Sci 1988;66:3010–6.

32. López-Gatius F. Side of gestation in dairy heifers affects subsequent sperm transport and pregnancy rates after deep insemination into one uterine horn. Theriogenology 1996;45:417–25.

33. Pursley JR. Deep uterine horn AI improves fertility of lactating dairy cows. J Dairy Sci 2004;87(Suppl. 1):372 (Abstr.).

34. Hawk HW, Tanabe TY. Effect of unilateral cornual insemination upon fertilization rate in superovulating and single-ovulating cattle. J Anim Sci 1986;63:551–60.

35. Williams BL, Gwazdauskas FC, Whittier WD, et al. Impact of site of inseminate deposition and environmental factors that influence reproduction of dairy cattle. J Dairy Sci 1988;71:2278–83.

36. McKenna T, Lenz RW, Fenton SE, et al. Nonreturn rates of dairy cattle following uterine body or cornual insemination. J Dairy Sci 1990;73:1779–83.

37. Diskin MG, Pursley JR, Kenny DA, et al. The effect of deep intrauterine placement of semen on conception rate in dairy cows. J Dairy Sci 2004;87(Suppl. 1):257 (Abstr.).

38. Gallagher GR, Senger PL. Concentrations of spermatozoa in the vagina of heifers after deposition of semen in the uterine horns, uterine body or cervix. J Reprod Fertil 1989;86:19–25.
39. Meirelles C, Kozicki LE, Weiss RR, et al. Comparison between deep intracornual artificial insemination (DIAI) and conventional artificial insemination (AI) using low concentration of spermatozoa in beef cattle. Braz Arch Biol Technol 2012;55(3): 371–4.
40. Carvalho PD, Souza AH, Dresch AR, et al. Placement of semen in uterine horns failed to improve fertilization rates in superovulated Holstein cows. J Dairy Sci 2012;95(Suppl. 2):575 (Abstr.).
41. Seidel GE Jr, Schenk JL, Herickhoff LA, et al. Insemination of heifers with sexed sperm. Theriogenology 1999;52:1407–20.
42. Seidel GE Jr, Schenk JL. Pregnancy rates in cattle with cryopreserved sexed sperm: Effects of sperm numbers per inseminate and site of sperm deposition. Anim Reprod Sci 2008;105(1–2):129–38.
43. Peters JL, Senger PL, Rosenberger JL, et al. Radiographic evaluation of bovine artificial inseminating technique among professional and herdsman-inseminators using .5- and .25-mL French straws. J Anim Sci 1984;59:1671–83.
44. Macpherson JW. Semen placement effects on fertility in bovines. J Dairy Sci 1968;51:807–8.
45. King J, Macpherson JW. Observations on retraining of artificial insemination technicians and its importance in maintaining efficiency. Can Vet Jour 1965;6(4):83–5.
46. Cembrowics HJ. Efficiency of inseminators. In: Proc.5th Int. Congr4. Anim. Reprod. Artif. Insem.; 1964. p. 624.
47. Graham E. The use a dye indicator for testing, training and evaluating technicians in artificial insemination. In: Proc. 1st Tech. Conf. Columbia, MO: AI and Bovine Reprod., National Association of Animal Breeders; 1966. p. 57–60.
48. Senger PL. Artificial insemination technique needs attention. In: Proc. 19th Ann. Conv. Louisville, KY: Amer. Assoc. Bovine Pract.; 1987. p. 114–6. https://doi.org/10.21423/aabppro19867580.

# Considerations for Using Natural Service with Estrous Synchronization Programs

George A. Perry, PhD

## KEYWORDS

- Bull fertility • Estrous synchronization • Natural service • Serving capacity

## KEY POINTS

- The major benefit of using estrous synchronization with natural service is getting cows to conceive early in the breeding season, specifically, giving them 2 chances to conceive within the first month of the breeding season.
- Pregnancy rates over a 28-day synchronized breeding season tended to be reduced when a bull-to-female ratio of 1:50 (77%) was used compared with a bull-to-female ratio of 1:16 (84%); however, no difference was detected between a bull-to-female ratio of 1:16 and 1:25 (83%).
- Pregnancy rates for synchronized females bred by natural service increased when females were serviced 2 or more times compared with when females were only serviced once.
- The most commonly used methods to assess male fertility and readiness for the breeding season is a breeding soundness examination.
- When single- versus multiple-sire use was compared in synchronized beef heifers (1:20 vs 2:40), mating performance and pregnancy rates were not different, but heifers in single-sire groups were serviced more times than those in multiple-sire groups.

## INTRODUCTION

Reproductive failure is a major source of economic loss in the beef industry. Most of this loss occurs because cows do not become pregnant during a defined breeding season. Therefore, the goal of any breeding program is to maximize the number of female cows that become pregnant, but of equal importance should be the timing of when females become pregnant. Timing has a large impact on profitability, as most beef operations market calves at weaning or shortly thereafter at local markets. Thus, the value of calves is based mostly on weight.

Estrous synchronization can benefit overall herd management. Cows that respond and conceive to a synchronized estrus have the following advantages: (1) exhibit

Texas A&M AgriLife Research and Extension Center, 1710 FM 3053 N, Overton, TX 75684, USA
*E-mail address:* George.Perry@ag.tamu.edu

Vet Clin Food Anim 40 (2024) 167–178
https://doi.org/10.1016/j.cvfa.2023.08.010
0749-0720/24/© 2023 Elsevier Inc. All rights reserved.

vetfood.theclinics.com

standing estrus at a predicted time, (2) conceive earlier in the breeding season, (3) calve earlier in the calving season, and (4) wean calves that are older and heavier. Some progestin-based estrous synchronization protocols can induce a proportion of anestrous cows to begin estrous cycles. This will decrease the anestrous postpartum interval and allow for additional opportunities for cows to conceive during a defined breeding season. A study conducted at Colorado State University indicated cows that conceived to a synchronized estrus calved on average 13 days earlier than cows that were not synchronized.[1] Although a successful breeding season relies on both female and male readiness, this review focuses on considerations for the male.

## THE BREEDING SOUNDNESS EXAMINATION

One of the most common methods to assess potential male fertility is a complete breeding soundness examination[2] (BSE; see Chapter 1: Bull Breeding Soundness Evaluation), which consists of an evaluation of semen quality, scrotal circumference, and physical fitness. A BSE is only effective when the bull being evaluated is postpubertal. Furthermore, the BSE only provides a snapshot of that bull's reproductive potential on that specific day, meaning that it cannot be reliably used to predict how the bull will continue to perform. This is largely due to the fact that sperm production is a continuous process, and the classification a bull receives at the completion of one BSE may differ from the classification that the same bull receives at the completion of a BSE performed at a later date.

### Minimum Requirements

The Society of Theriogenology[3] indicates that in order for bulls to pass a BSE they must have obtained a minimum scrotal circumference based on their age, exhibit greater than 30% progressive motility, and have at least 70% morphologically normal sperm. Bulls meeting these minimum requirements are classified as *satisfactory potential breeders*. When the minimum requirements are not met, the bull will be classified as either *deferred* (indicating that the bull should be tested again at a later date) or an *unsatisfactory potential breeder* (suggesting the bull should be culled). These examinations should occur approximately 8 weeks before the start of the breeding season, as this will allow time for deferred bulls to be retested or to find a replacement herd bull. Bulls that are classified as *satisfactory potential breeders* should be monitored to make sure they are not injured or experience a decrease in nutrition, as these can cause changes in semen quality before the start of the breeding season.

### Impacts on Fertility

As scrotal circumference increases, the production of high-quality sperm will also increase.[4,5] Scrotal circumference is a highly heritable trait,[6–9] as bulls with a larger scrotal circumference will sire sons with a larger scrotal circumference.[10] Furthermore, bulls with a larger scrotal circumference sire daughters that achieve puberty at an earlier age[10] and are more likely to become pregnant earlier.[11]

Semen quality can be impacted by several factors, and sperm cell morphology is the most common reason a bull is not classified as a satisfactory potential breeder when using the BSE standards established by the Society for Theriogenology.[12] The most common factors that can impact sperm production are injury, disease, fever,[13] and extreme environmental conditions.[14–16] Thus, if a bull is injured, stressed, or experiences extreme environmental conditions before or during the breeding season, a precautionary step may be to perform a BSE or add an additional sire to the breeding group to prevent low pregnancy rates owing to the hindered sperm production/quality of the first sire.

## LIMITATIONS TO NATURAL SERVICE IN A SYNCHRONIZATION PROGRAM
### Inseminator Efficiency

With natural service, inseminator efficiency is not typically considered an issue, as the bull should breed the cow. The purpose of the physical examination portion of a BSE is to determine a bull's mating ability. Mating ability can be described as the physical capabilities needed to successfully breed a cow. In addition to structural unsoundness, diseases or injuries to the penis or prepuce can result in an inability to breed via natural service. These abnormalities will only be detected by careful examination or observing an attempted mating of a cow. A bull that has high-quality semen but is unable to physically breed cows is unsatisfactory for natural service.

Satisfactory potential breeders should be of good health and appropriate body condition at the start of the breeding season (BCS of 6–7 on a 1–9 scale). This will ensure that as the bull progresses through the breeding season and begins to lose weight, the reserves that are being lost are fat and not muscle. Bulls that are not of appropriate fitness may experience a reduction in libido or fertility. A herd bull's vision should not be impaired, as vision is essential to recognize estrus behavior. Structurally, a bull should be sound and capable of supporting his weight on his hind legs and feet when mounting a female.[2]

### Libido

Libido, or the desire/willingness to mate, has a positive effect on pregnancy rates to natural service; however, libido is not commonly measured. Scrotal circumference, semen quality, and mating ability are not correlated to libido,[17,18] so although a bull may be classified as a satisfactory potential breeder, his libido could be low. Observing bulls when they are exposed to estrual females could be advantageous to producers, especially in single-sire pastures. Several studies have indicated libido has a significant genetic component[19–21] and is considered to be a moderately heritable (0.59) trait.[19]

### Social Effects

When using multiple-sire breeding pastures, social dominance should be taken into consideration when deciding which bulls to pair together. Social rankings exist among bulls and thus may influence the number of females a particular sire is willing/able to breed (**Table 1**).[22] Thus, producers should pay special attention to sires that have decreased semen quality (smaller scrotal circumference, borderline motility and morphology) but are socially dominant, as this dominance could prevent a more fertile, but less dominant bull from being able to breed as many females. When multiple cows are in estrus at the same time, they form a sexually active group. This grouping together increases the ability of a dominant (but possibly less fertile) bull to keep subordinate bulls from breeding cows. When single- versus multiple-sire use was compared in synchronized beef heifers (1:20 vs 2:40), mating performance of bulls and pregnancy rates were not different, but heifers in single-sire herds were serviced more times than those in multiple-sire herds (4.1 ± 0.6 vs 2.6 ± 0.2),[23] and pregnancy rates increased when females were serviced 2 or more times compared with females only serviced once.[24]

A bull's seniority is the major factor influencing his social ranking, with the dominant bull in a breeding cadre likely being an older bull.[25] Therefore, it is important not to

**Table 1**
**Percent calf crop sired by individual sires in multiple-sire pastures[22]**

| | Percent Calf Crop Sired | | | | |
|---|---|---|---|---|---|
| Social Rank | Pasture 1 | Pasture 2 | Pasture 3 | Pasture 4 | Pasture 5 |
| Bull 1 | 30% | 34% | 44% | 92% | 75% |
| Bull 2 | 21% | 29% | 18% | 3% | 25% |
| Bull 3 | 12% | 21% | 16% | 3% | 0% |
| Bull 4 | 10% | 6% | 4% | | |
| Bull 5 | 9% | 4% | 4% | | |
| Bull 6 | 9% | 1% | 4% | | |
| Bull 7 | 5% | 1% | 2% | | |
| Bull 8 | | | 2% | | |
| Bull 9 | | | 2% | | |
| Bull 10 | | | 0% | | |
| Number of calves born | 73 | 64 | 43 | 28 | 32 |

introduce a young (yearling) bull into a herd with older, more mature bulls. This can be avoided by separating cows into single-sire breeding groups. In multiple-sire breeding groups, multiple bulls tend to breed the same sexually responsive females.[23] This leads to females being bred by more than one bull and increases the risk of injury to a bull. Sire age also influences the efficiency of bulls when placed with synchronized females. When bulls (1–7 years of age) were used at a ratio of 1:7 to 1:51, yearling bulls had the lowest pregnancy rates ($30.2 \pm 5.1\%$, based on number of females exhibiting estrus) compared with 2-year-old ($40.3 \pm 6.0\%$) and mature bulls (3 years and older; $50.7 \pm 4.5\%$), even though pregnancy rate was not affected by bull-to-female ratio or number of females exhibiting estrus.[24]

*Bull-to-Female Ratio*

When cows are bred by natural service, the time required to detect estrus is not a concern because a bull with good libido will detect cows that are in standing estrus, but the serving capacity of the bull becomes a critical management consideration. Recommendations for the bull-to-female ratio in a nonsynchronized herd range from 1:10 to 1:60. No differences were detected between a bull-to-female ratio of 1:25 and 1:60 for estrus detection or pregnancy rates in the first 21 days of the breeding season.[26] When cows are synchronized and bred by natural service, management considerations should be made for the serving capacity of the bull. Healy and coworkers[27] reported a tendency ($P<.10$) for pregnancy rates to be reduced over a 28-day synchronized breeding season when a bull-to-female ratio of 1:50 (77%) was used compared with a ratio of 1:16 (84%); however, no difference was detected between a bull-to-female ratio of 1:16 and 1:25 (84% and 83%, respectively). Overall, bull-to-female ratios will vary depending on the reproductive capacity of an individual bull. Ratios can be increased in single-sire breeding groups, but bulls should be observed during the breeding season to be sure bulls continue to be capable of mating. Poor performance of a bull in a single-sire breeding group will affect the entire calf crop of that group. Also remember, yearling bulls have a decreased serving capacity compared with 2 -year-old bulls, and bulls that are 3 years old and older have the greatest serving capacity.[24] Therefore, it is important to remember that young bulls should be used at a lower bull-to-female ratio than older bulls.

In a free-range condition, dairy bulls serviced a female 3 to 10 times during estrus.[28] Similarly, with synchronized females, beef bulls averaged 55 services (range of 14–101) during a 30-hour period of time,[29] and services per female averaged 3 (range 1–13) when bull-to-female ratios were 1:10 to 1:35.[30] With these increased number of services per cow, does the number of sperm in successive ejaculates decrease, and is there an impact on fertility? Although the answer to these questions is not exactly known, it has been reported that Holstein bulls can produce approximately $5 \times 10^6$ sperm per minute[28] with the average ejaculate containing 4.8 billion sperm.[31] Collection of 4 Holstein bulls revealed that volume of an ejaculate decreased from the first 2 ejaculates to the third to seventh ejaculate and further decreased in later ejaculates (8 to 14), but concentration of sperm per milliliter was not significantly different between the third and fourth ejaculate ($470 \times 10^6$ per milliliter) and the eleventh to fourteenth ejaculate ($232 \times 10^6$ per milliliter).[32] Therefore, the number of sperm in an ejaculate is likely not the limiting factor with natural service, and when females were synchronized, there was a linear increase in pregnancy rates as number of services increased.[30]

## SELECTION OF PROTOCOLS

Similar to synchronization with artificial insemination (AI), the benefits of synchronization with natural service is not only increasing conception rates early in the breeding season, but more importantly, providing 2 chances to conceive within the first month of the breeding season. Unlike synchronization for AI whereby the goal is to increase the number of females in estrus in the shortest period of time, synchronization for natural service must consider the limitations of natural service (serving capacity of the bull). Thus, a protocol that distributes estrus over a period of at least 10 days is more advantageous for natural service. Therefore, it is necessary to understand how different synchronization products work with the physiology of the estrous cycle.

Prostaglandin $F_{2\alpha}$ (PG) is a naturally occurring hormone that regresses the corpus luteum (CL) and allows cows to return to standing estrus.[33–35] Administering PG will cause regression of a CL before it would normally regress on its own and allows for control of the luteal phase of the estrous cycle. During the first 5 days of luteal development, the CL is not responsive to PG,[33,35] but when administered during the responsive period (days 5–17), the CL will regress, and the animal will exhibit standing estrus 48 to 120 hours after administration.[36] If an animal does not have a CL present (cows in the postpartum anestrous period or heifers that have not reached puberty), they will not respond to administration of PG. Therefore, animals must be cycling, and be between days 5 and 17 of the estrous cycle to respond to PG.

Progestins mimic the progesterone produced by the CL to inhibit ovulation and have been reported to be an effective method of synchronizing ovulation in cattle.[37] Progestins control the estrous cycle by extending the luteal phase, inhibiting ovulation after natural regression of the CL, and preventing standing estrus and ovulation. Following the removal of the progestin, progesterone concentrations decrease, and standing estrus and ovulation will occur. Thus, by inhibiting estrus for 7 days, the normal 21-day estrous cycle of a herd is reduced to 14 days. However, when a CL regresses and cows are exposed to a progestin to inhibit ovulation of the dominant follicle, the follicle will continue to grow and will become a persistent follicle. Breeding animals at the first estrus after exposure for more than 7 days to a progestin results in decreased fertility,[38,39] but subsequent ovulations will have normal fertility.[37]

### The Anestrous Period

Anestrus occurs when an animal does not exhibit normal estrous cycles. This occurs in heifers before they reach puberty and in cows following parturition (calving). During an anestrous period, normal follicular waves occur, but standing estrus and ovulation do not occur. Therefore, during the anestrous period, heifers/cows cannot become pregnant. Thus, the anestrous postpartum interval is a major contributing factor to cows failing to become pregnant and calving on a yearly interval.[40,41] However, treatment with progestins (ie, progesterone or melengestrol acetate, MGA) can induce ovulation in anestrous postpartum cows,[42–44] thereby shortening the anestrous postpartum interval.

In a small study, peripubertal heifers treated with MGA (an orally active progestin) for 10 days resulted in a similar number of MGA-treated heifers and control heifers attaining puberty by day 7 after MGA withdrawal; however, by day 10 after MGA withdrawal, 50% more of the treated heifers attained puberty compared with the control heifers.[45] Synchronization with a progestin resulted in more ($P<.01$) heifers becoming pregnant (67% and 62%) during the first 7 days of the breeding season compared with non-synchronized heifers (23%).[46] When a controlled internal drug-releasing device (CIDR) containing progesterone was inserted 7 days before the start of the breeding season and removed the day the bull was introduced (no injections), more CIDR-treated cows ($P<.05$; 43%) became pregnant by day 10 compared with nonsynchronized cows (35%).[47] However, when a single injection of PG was administered to a group of anestrous cows, no difference was detected between treated and nontreated cows (13.6% and 22.7%, respectively).[48] Therefore, progestin-based estrous synchronization protocols capable of inducing puberty and shortening the anestrous postpartum period can result in an even greater percentage of cows having a chance to become pregnant during the first few days of the breeding season.

Not all progestins are equally effective at inducing estrous cycles in anestrous postpartum cows. Evidence for this difference is based on differences in the ability of progesterone (CIDR) and MGA to induce ovulation in anestrous cows (**Fig. 1**). Fewer anestrous cows treated with MGA (0.5 mg MGA•cow$^{-1}$•d$^{-1}$ for 7 days) ovulated within 6 days of progestin removal compared with progesterone-treated (1.9 g of progesterone contained in a CIDR for 6 days) cows (33% and 91%, respectively),[44] and a decreased number of control cows (cows that spontaneously initiated estrous cycles;

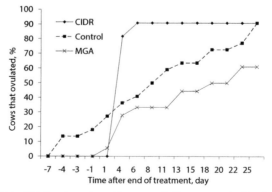

**Fig. 1.** Effect of progestin treatment on the cumulative percent of animals that had ovulated by day of treatment (day 0 = last day of feeding MGA, and day of CIDR removal). Control animals received no treatment. Treatment, $P<.01$; day, $P<.01$; treatment × day, $P<.01$.[44]

23%) or MGA-treated anestrous cows (46%) exhibited normal length luteal phases compared with progesterone-treated cows (100%).[44,49] However, by day 22 after treatment withdrawal, no difference was detected ($P>.05$) between the percentage of CIDR-treated cows that had ovulated (91%) and the percentage of MGA-treated cows that had ovulated (61%; see **Fig. 1**).[44]

### Success of Selected Protocols

In the following studies, a bull-to-female ratio of up to 1:25 was used. A single injection of PG on day 5 of the breeding season (**Fig. 2**) resulted in more cycling cows becoming pregnant during days 5 to 9 of the breeding season compared with cycling cows not treated with PG (55.7% vs 25.0% respectively).[48] Pregnancy rates were similar ($P>.10$) for cows in which estrus was synchronized with a single injection of PG and exposed to a bull for 80 hours compared with nonsynchronized cows exposed to a bull for 21 days.[50] When cows were synchronized with a single injection of PG on day 5 of the breeding season, there were no differences in pregnancy rates over the first 25 days of the breeding season (1 cycle) between synchronized and nonsynchronized cows.[48] Among dairy cattle, PG has been used for synchronization with natural service by administering 2 injections of PG 14 days apart and introducing bulls 14 days after the second injection. When this method was compared with a fixed-time AI protocol, there was no difference in the overall 21-day pregnancy rate between the 2

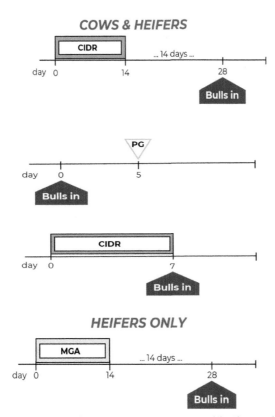

**Fig. 2.** Recommended protocols for synchronizing cows and heifers to be bred by natural service.

**Table 2**
Comparison between synchronized and nonsynchronized pregnancy rates when bred by natural service in cows and heifers

| Study | Period of Bull Exposure | Cows/Heifers | Synchronization Method | Pregnancy Rate Anestrual / Unknown | Estrual |
|---|---|---|---|---|---|
| Whittier et al,[48] 1991 | 4 d | | 1 shot PG | 13.6% | 55.7%[a] |
| | | Cows | Not synchronized | 22.7% | 25.0%[b] |
| Lamb et al,[47] 2008 | 10 d | | CIDR | 43%[a] | |
| | | Cows | Not synchronized | 35%[c] | |
| Landivar et al,[50] 1985 | 80 h | | 1 shot PG | 19% | |
| | 21 d | Cows | Not synchronized | 33% | |
| Whittier et al,[48] 1991 | 25 d | | 1 shot PG | 59.1% | |
| | 21 d | Cows | Not synchronized | 59.1% | |
| Lamb et al,[47] 2008 | 30 d | | CIDR | 64.4% | 86.1% |
| | | Cows | Not synchronized | 64.7% | 76.3% |
| Locke et al,[52] 2020 | 21 d | | 14-d CIDR | 52% | 55% |
| | | Heifers | 14-d MGA | 53% | 59% |
| Locke et al,[52] 2020 | 61 d | | 14-d CIDR | 57% | 80% |
| | | Heifers | 14-d MGA | 66% | 90% |

Pregnancy rates within a study and estrous cycling status having different superscripts are different
[a,b]$P<.01$; [a,c]$P<.05$.

treatments, but the daily rate of pregnancy was increased in the natural service group compared with the fixed-time AI group.[51] Therefore, the greatest benefit of estrous synchronization with natural service is the ability to increase pregnancy rates during the first week of the breeding season (**Table 2**) and thus increase the number of calves that are born at the start of the calving season.

The ability to induce estrous cycles with a progestin has also been tested with natural service. A CIDR was inserted for 7 days and removed the day bulls were introduced to cows (no injections were given; see **Fig. 2**).[47] The use of a CIDR to synchronize with natural service decreased the average days to conception and also increased the percentage of animals that conceived in the first 10 days of the breeding season (35.9% vs 30.8%).[47] Pregnancy rates over the first 30 days of the breeding season did not differ between females treated with a CIDR and controls (68.2% vs 66.7%, respectively).[47]

Long-term progestin exposure has also been used to successfully synchronize females for natural service[52]; however, care should be taken when using a long-term progestin protocol. When using a long-term progestin protocol and progestin is administered after the CL regresses, a persistent follicle will form. Breeding animals at the first estrus/ovulation after long-term progestin exposure will have decreased fertility,[38,39] but subsequent ovulations will have normal fertility.[37] Thus, after feeding MGA (heifers only) or inserting a CIDR for 14 days, it is recommended that females not be exposed to natural service for 14 days after progestin removal (see **Fig. 2**).

## SUMMARY

Estrous synchronization provides the benefit of more females conceiving early in the breeding season and giving females that do not conceive to the first service an opportunity for a second service within the first 30 days of the breeding season. When cows are synchronized, the number of animals that exhibit estrus in a short period of time increases, and considerations need to be made to ensure a bull is fertile and can cover as many females as possible. A BSE is the most common method to determine if a bull is producing fertile semen. With synchronized females, it is important to remember that mature bulls (3 years old or older) have increased efficiency in getting cows pregnant compared with younger bulls. The use of multiple sires in a pasture offers some protection if a bull gets injured, but in multisire pastures, social dominance may lead to one sire breeding most cows. When single- versus multiple-sire systems were compared, mating performance and pregnancy rates did not differ, but heifers in single-sire groups were serviced more times than those in multiple-sire groups. Pregnancy rates increased when females were serviced 2 or more times compared with females only serviced once. No difference was detected in pregnancy rates between a bull-to-female ratio of 1:16 and 1:25, but pregnancy rates tended to decrease at a ratio of 1:50. Consideration should also be given to the selection of the protocol that is used. A protocol that distributes estrus over 10 to 14 days is ideal to not over-work a bull. When a protocol that is recommended for natural service is used, and mature, fertile bulls are placed with the estrous synchronized females, a successful breeding season with a large proportion of the herd conceiving early in the breeding season will likely be achieved.

## CLINICS CARE POINTS

- Make sure bulls have passed a breeding soundness examination before using them in a synchronized breeding season.
- Use a synchronization protocol that distributes estrus over a period of at least 10 day when using natural service.
- With synchronized females, it is important to remember that mature bulls (3 years old or older) have increased efficiency in getting cows pregnant compared with younger bulls.

## DISCLSOURE

The author has no relationship with any commerical company that has a direct financial interest in the subject matter.

## FUNDING

Our research our the years has primarily been supported multistate Hatch funds (project #9835), the U.S. National Insitiute of Food and Agriculture, and the National Science Foundation.

## REFERENCES

1. Schafer DW, Brinks JS, LeFever DG. Increased calf weaning weight and weight via estrus synchronization, In: *Beef program report.* Ft. Collins, CO: Colorado State University; 1990. p. 115–24.
2. Koziol JH, Armstrong CL. Manual for breeding soundness examination of bulls. 2nd edition. Providence, RI: Society for Theriogenology; 2018.
3. Chenoweth PJ, Spitzer JC, Hopkins FM. A new bull breeding soundness evaluation form. San Antonio, TX: Paper presented at: Proc. Ann. Mtng. Soc. for Theriogenology; 1992.

4. Foote RH, Seidel GE Jr, Hahn J, et al. Seminal quality, spermatozoal outpost, and testicular changes in growing Holstein bulls. J Dairy Sci 1977;60(1):85–8.

5. Gipson TA, Vogt DW, Massey JW, et al. Associations of scrotal circumference with semen traits in young beef bulls. Theriogenology 1985;24(2):217–25.

6. Coulter GH, Rounsaville TR, Foote RH. Heritability of testicular size and consistency in Holstein bulls. J Anim Sci 1976;43(1):9–12.

7. Smith BA, Brinks JS, Richardson GV. Estimation of genetic parameters among breeding soundness examination components and growth traits in yearling bulls. J Anim Sci 1989;67(11):2892–6.

8. Boligon AA, Baldi F, de Albuquerque LG. Genetic parameters and relationships between growth traits and scrotal circumference measured at different ages in Nellore cattle. Genet Mol Biol 2011;34(2):225–30.

9. Knights SA, Baker RL, Gianola D, et al. Estimates of heritabilities and of genetic and phenotypic correlations among growth and reproductive traits in yearling Angus bulls. J Anim Sci 1984;58(4):887–93.

10. Smith BA, Brinks JS, Richardson GV. Relationships of sire scrotal circumference to offspring reproduction and growth. J Anim Sci 1989;67(11):2881–5.

11. Toelle VD, Robison OW. Estimates of genetic correlations between testicular measurements and female reproductive traits in cattle. J Anim Sci 1985;60(1):89–100.

12. Carson RL, Wenzel JG. Observations using the new bull-breeding soundness evaluation forms in adult and young bulls. Vet Clin North Am Food Anim Pract 1997;13(2):305–11.

13. Coulter GH. Beef bull fertility: factors affecting seminal quality. In: Fields MJ, Sands RS, editors. Factors affecting calf crop. Ann Arbor, MI: CRC Press; 1994. p. 307–17.

14. Casady RB, Meyers RM, Legates JE. The effect of exposure to high ambient temperature on spermatogenesis in the dairy bull. J Dairy Sci 1953;36:14.

15. Skinner JD, Louw GN. Heat stress and spermatogenesis in Bos indicus and Bos taurus cattle. J Appl Physiol 1966;21(6):1784–90.

16. Meyerhoeffer DC, Wettemann RP, Coleman SW, et al. Reproductive criteria of beef bulls during and after exposure to increased ambient temperature. J Anim Sci 1985;60(2):352–7.

17. Blockey MA. Studies on the social and sexual behavior of bulls. Victoria, Australia: University of Melbourne; 1975.

18. Chenoweth PJ, Abbitt B, McInerney MJ. Libido, serving capacity and breeding soundness in beef bulls. Stn CSUE 1977;966:918.

19. Blockey MA. Relationship between serving capacity of beef bulls as predicted by the yard test and their fertility during paddock mating. Aust Vet J 1989;66(11):348–51.

20. Boyd GW, Lunstra DD, Corah LR. Serving capacity of crossbred yearling beef bulls. I. Single-sire mating behavior and fertility during average and heavy mating loads at pasture. J Anim Sci 1989;67(1):60–71.

21. Chenoweth PJ. Libido and mating behavior in bulls, boars and rams. A review. Theriogenology 1981;16(2):155–77.

22. Lehrer AR, Brown MB, Schindler H, et al. Paternity tests in multisired beef herds by blood grouping. Acta Vet Scand 1977;18(4):433–41.

23. Farin PW, Chenoweth PJ, Mateos ER, et al. Beef bulls mated to estrus synchronized heifers: Single- vs multi-sire breeding groups. Theriogenology 1982; 17(4):365–72.

24. Pexton JE, Farin PW, Rupp GP, et al. Factors affecting mating activity and pregnancy rates with beef bulls mated to estrus synchronized females. Theriogenology 1990;34(6):1059–70.

25. Chenoweth PJ. Bull libido/serving capacity. Vet Clin Food Anim Pract 1997;13: 331–44.

26. Rupp GP, Ball L, Shoop MC, et al. Reproductive efficiency of bulls in natural service: effects of male to female ratio and single- vs multiple-sire breeding groups. J Am Vet Med Assoc 1977;171(7):639–42.

27. Healy VM, Boyd GW, Gutierrez PH, et al. Investigating optimal bull:heifer ratios required for estrus-synchronized heifers. J Anim Sci 1993;71(2):291–7.

28. Chenoweth PJ. Sexual behavior of the bull: a review. J Dairy Sci 1983;66(1): 173–9.

29. Farin PW, Pexton JE, Chenoweth PJ, et al. Libido, service capacity and mating performance of bulls breeding synchronized heifers. J Anim Sci 1978;359. abstr.

30. Farin PW. Sexual behavior and fertility in beef bulls. Ft. Collins, CO: Colorado State University; 1980.

31. Hafs HD, Hoyt RS, Bratton RW. Libido, Sperm Characteristics, Sperm Output, and Fertility of Mature Dairy Bulls Ejaculated Daily or Weekly for Thirty-Two Weeks. J Dairy Sci 1959;42(4):626–36.

32. Bame JH. Effect of extra-gonadal sperm depletion on steroid hormone profiles in semen of bulls. Virginia Tech: Dairy Science; 1983.

33. Rowson LE, Tervit R, Brand A. The use of prostaglandins for synchronization of oestrus in cattle. J Reprod Fertil 1972;29(1):145.

34. Tervit HR, Rowson LE, Brand A. Synchronization of oestrus in cattle using a prostaglandin F2alpha analogue (ICI 79939). J Reprod Fertil 1973;34(1):179–81.

35. Lauderdale JW. Effects of PGF2a on pregnancy and estrous cycle of cattle. J Anim Sci 1972;35:246, abstr.

36. Lauderdale JW, Seguin BE, Stellflug JN, et al. Fertility of cattle following PGF2 alpha injection. J Anim Sci 1974;38(5):964–7.

37. Odde KG. A review of synchronization of estrus in postpartum cattle. J Anim Sci 1990;68(3):817–30.

38. Ahmad N, Schrick FN, Butcher RL, et al. Effect of persistent follicles on early embryonic losses in beef cows. Biol Reprod 1995;52(5):1129–35.

39. Mihm M, Baguisi A, Boland MP, et al. Association between the duration of dominance of the ovulatory follicle and pregnancy rate in beef heifers. J Reprod Fertil 1994;102(1):123–30.

40. Short RE, Bellows RA, Staigmiller RB, et al. Physiological mechanisms controlling anestrus and infertility in postpartum beef cattle. J Anim Sci 1990;68(3):799–816.

41. Yavas Y, Walton JS. Postpartum acyclicity in suckled beef cows: a review. Theriogenology 2000;54(1):25–55.

42. Yavas Y, Walton JS. Induction of ovulation in postpartum suckled beef cows: a review. Theriogenology 2000;54(1):1–23.

43. Lucy MC, Billings HJ, Butler WR, et al. Efficacy of an intravaginal progesterone insert and an injection of $PGF_{2\alpha}$ for synchronizing estrus and shortening the interval to pregnancy in postpartum beef cows, peripubertal beef heifers, and dairy heifers. J Anim Sci 2001;79(4):982–95.

44. Perry GA, Smith MF, Geary TW. Ability of intravaginal progesterone inserts and melengestrol acetate to induce estrous cycles in postpartum beef cows. J Anim Sci 2004;82(3):695–704.

45. Imwalle DB, Patterson DJ, Schillo KK. Effects of melengestrol acetate on onset of puberty, follicular growth, and patterns of luteinizing hormone secretion in beef heifers. Biol Reprod 1998;58(6):1432–6.

46. Plugge BL, Deutscher GH, Davis RL. Comparison of melengestrol acetate (MGA) and lutalyse combination to Syncro-mate B (SMB) in estrous synchronization programs utilizing AI or natural service. J Anim Sci 1989;67(Suppl. 2):87.

47. Lamb GC, Dahlen CR, Vonnahme KA, et al. Influence of a CIDR prior to bull breeding on pregnancy rates and subsequent calving distribution. Anim Reprod Sci 2008;108(3–4):269–78.

48. Whittier JC, Caldwell RW, Anthony RV, et al. Effect of a prostaglandin F2 alpha injection 96 hours after introduction of intact bulls on estrus and calving distribution of beef cows. J Anim Sci 1991;69(12):4670–7.

49. Smith VG, Chenault JR, McAllister JF, et al. Response of postpartum beef cows to exogenous progestogens and gonadotropin releasing hormone. J Anim Sci 1987; 64(2):540–51.

50. Landivar C, Galina CS, Duchateau A, et al. Fertility trial in Zebu cattle after a natural or controlled estrus with prostaglandin F2 Alpha, comparing natural mating with artificial insemination. Theriogenology 1985;23(3):421–9.

51. Lima FS, Risco CA, Thatcher MJ, et al. Comparison of reproductive performance in lactating dairy cows bred by natural service or timed artificial insemination. J Dairy Sci 2009;92(11):5456–66.

52. Locke JWC, Thomas JM, Knickmeyer ER, et al. Comparison of long-term progestin-based protocols to synchronize estrus prior to natural service or fixed-time artificial insemination in Bos indicus-influenced beef heifers. Anim Reprod Sci 2020;218:106475.

# Managing Beef Bulls During the Off-Season

Arthur Lee Jones, DVM, MS

## KEYWORDS

- Bull management • Bull housing • Social dominance • Nutrition

## KEY POINTS

- Proper management of herd bulls during the nonbreeding season is essential for peak performance of bulls in subsequent breeding season.
- Routine herd health practices should be performed at least 60 days before introducing bulls with the cows.
- Adequate nutrition during the nonbreeding period allows bulls to replace lost condition during the breeding season and prepare for optimum performance in the upcoming breeding season.
- Overconditioned bulls may be a higher risk of injury and lameness, as well as have unsatisfactory breeding soundness examination classification.

## INTRODUCTION

As approximately 94% of beef cow-calf operations only use natural service for breeding their cows and heifers,[1] replacement bulls are a significant, necessary cost of producing beef calves. The value realized from beef bulls includes number and quality of calves sired, weight of calves sold, production value of daughters retained, and the bull's salvage value. Considering the importance of maintaining and recouping the cost of this significant investment, there is little information in peer reviewed literature about maintaining bulls in the off-season to prepare the bull for optimum performance in subsequent breeding seasons. As the costs of good quality beef bulls can easily exceed $3000 to 5000, maintaining herd bulls to be healthy, physically sound, and fertile for future breeding seasons is vital. Therefore, it is equally important to identify or recognize risk factors that could predispose bulls to culling due to unsatisfactory breeding soundness examination (BSE) classification, lameness, or other health events.

According to a 2017 USDA survey,[1] of the beef operations that had a controlled breeding season, greater than 90% had a season less than 150 days. Therefore, many beef bulls are housed separately from the breeding herd for most of the year.

Senior Professional Services Veterinarian - Beef, Boehringer-Ingelheim Animal Health, 3239 Satellite Boulevard, Duluth, GA 30096, USA
*E-mail address:* leejones@uga.edu

Vet Clin Food Anim 40 (2024) 179–183
https://doi.org/10.1016/j.cvfa.2023.09.004
0749-0720/24/© 2023 Elsevier Inc. All rights reserved.

Maintaining bulls is just as important as the decision to purchase one. Bulls need optimum off-season management so they perform best during the following season. Operations that do not properly care for their bulls take a chance that the bull might not be fit for the next breeding season. The bull needs to be ready to breed cows the first day they are returned to the herd so a good off-season plan is essential for top performance. This plan needs to consider the age of the bull(s), natural bull behavior, nutritional status, space and environment, and health program.

## INTRODUCING BULLS TO THE BULL PASTURE: SOCIAL DOMINANCE

Gathering bulls at the end of breeding season on large operations using multiple pastures may take several days, whereas smaller operations might be able to accomplish the task in 1 or 2 days. It is natural for bulls to fight to establish social hierarchy. Removing them from a structured herd situation and introducing them together disrupts the previously established hierarchy. Ideally, it is best to introduce all bulls that will share an off-season pasture in their pasture at the same time. This is difficult when gathering bulls from breeding herds over several days. When logistically feasible, holding bulls in temporary pens before commingling is ideal to reduce fighting.[2] Continually introducing bulls over the course of days or weeks increases the amount of time the bulls will be fighting and increases the odds one will get hurt. Seniority, age, size, and stamina determine social ranking of bulls and seems to extend into the breeding pasture among bulls housed together.[3] To reduce fighting, anecdotal reports describe pouring apple cider vinegar on bulls before introduction or putting a male goat or a donkey in the bull pen.[4] Some donkeys will intervene when bulls start fighting. No controlled studies have been published on these tactics and according to extension articles the results have been mixed.[4]

It is better to keep young bulls separate from older, bigger bulls.[2,3,5] Younger and smaller bulls could be injured if fighting occurs. As social dominance extends from the "bull pen" to the breeding herd, the younger, smaller subordinate bulls may not breed as many cows as the dominant bull when placed in the same breeding pasture.[3]

Evaluation of hooves and legs is also important at the end of the breeding season (see Joe C. Paschal and Arthur Lee Jones's article, "Physical Evaluation of Beef Bulls," in this issue.). Bulls that are old, lame, have bad hooves, or have some other physical problem like a bad eye or injury may need to be culled.[6,7] In a survey among California producers evaluating beef bull management, bull age, structural soundness, injury, and fertility were the top reasons for culling bulls.[8] Although trimming can alleviate some hoof problems, some hoof problems are hereditary. Therefore, it is advisable to either cull the bull or use him as a terminal breeder and not keep his offspring as replacements. Inspecting for corns or other hoof problems and correcting those issues in the off-season helps ensure the bull will be functional for the next season. A thorough examination of hoof conformation is also part of the BSE. Evaluating expected progeny differences associated with foot quality (ie, claw set and foot angle for registered Angus bulls) before purchasing a bull can also help producers minimize hoof structural issues. Procedures such as hoof trimming or other lameness treatment, as well as BSE, should be performed well in advance of the breeding season to allow adequate recovery before exposure to the breeding herd.[2,5] This may also be an ideal time for herd vaccinations to limit the frequency of handling and potential injury.

## ENVIRONMENT

Low stress environment is important. Making sure bulls have plenty of space to avoid each other also helps reduce injuries from fighting as bulls kept in close quarters have a tendency to fight more often. Adequate shelter for the region is also a significant consideration. Bulls exposed to extremely low temperatures and windy conditions may suffer from severe frostbite to the scrotum and testicles or epididymis and be at risk for an unsatisfactory BSE classification.[7,9] Alternatively, bulls exposed to extreme hot and humid conditions can have suboptimal thermoregulation of the testis, disrupting spermatogenesis and semen quality.[10]

Bulls are destructive. They can tear up anything, sometimes out of boredom. Hay feeders or bunks, mineral feeders or anything else needs to be tough enough for bulls. If bulls bend or break metal feeders, the sharp pieces or edges could possibly injure a bull. It is important to make sure all the equipment in their pasture is "bull proof" and inspected often.

## NUTRITION

Keeping younger and smaller bulls separate from larger bulls also provides an opportunity to feed any young bulls that might have lost a lot of condition during their first breeding season.[2,5,7] Similar to first-calf heifers, young bulls are still growing and have greater nutritional requirements compared with mature bulls. Therefore, young bulls should not need to compete with older bulls for nutrition. If space allows, separate pastures facilitate more optimum management.[2,5,7] While young, growing bulls need more nutrition, the older bulls do not need to get too fat.[6,9] Using body condition scores of 1 to 9, optimal condition is a body condition score of 5 to 6.[7] Under- or over-conditioned bulls are at risk of having an unsatisfactory BSE.[9] Moreover, over conditioned bulls are also at risk of developing musculoskeletal problems. A good nutrition program includes adequate minerals. One bag of minerals typically provides 200 feedings (4 oz/head/day). If there are not enough bulls in a pasture to consume the mineral to keep it fresh or from getting wet it is better to only put enough in the mineral feeder for 2 weeks at the time. A high-quality mineral program is crucial for optimum future fertility.[2,7,11] Access to clean, fresh water is also important.

## HERD HEALTH

It is generally recommended that bulls be on the same vaccination program as the cow herd.[5,7] It is more convenient to vaccinate at the time that BSEs are done but some producers may prefer to vaccinate the bulls after bringing them home. It is important that the vaccine protects against *Bovine viral diarrhea virus* 1 and 2, *Infectious Bovine Rhinotracheitis*, *Bovine respiratory syncytial virus*, and leptospirosis.[5,6] Vibrio (*Camplylobacter fetus venerealis*, *Cfv*) may also be important if vibrio has been diagnosed on the farm.[5] Cows are exposed to vibrio when bred by infected bulls. Vaccination for *Cfv* may be especially important if bulls are in large, extensive pastures, which is common in some states in the Western United States. The primary method of trichomoniasis control is testing and culling infected bulls and open cows. Some studies have shown that vaccination of young bulls can prevent infection in experimentally challenged bulls[12,13] but vaccination did not clear already infected bulls.[14]

Although older bulls may be resistant to internal parasites, they do need lice and fly control. If bulls are scratching due to lice, they can be destructive on fence posts, buildings, and equipment. Feed through fly control or fly tags and pour-on products for lice control are important. Remote insecticide applicators project insecticide-filled gel capsules that burst on impact to control flies and lice, and allow producers to periodically apply insecticide as needed. These have an advantage of not having to risk injury of gathering and working bulls through a chute or alley to apply the insecticide. Bulls can attract a lot of flies, so control is important. There have been lay articles that suggested some pour-on products may reduce bull fertility. Trials have shown no detrimental effect of the currently approved pour-on or injectable products on bull fertility when used at their label dose.[15]

## BIOSECURITY AND TESTING

If the ranch is an endemic area for trichomoniasis, testing bulls for trichomoniasis is best done after they have been out of the herd for at least 3 weeks. Testing for *Tritrichomonas foetus* and/or Cfv can also be done at the same time (see Arthur Lee Jones's article, "Sexually Transmitted Diseases of Bulls" in this issue.) as the BSE. The BSE procedure is described in (see Arthur E. Heath King and Richard M. Hopper's article, "The Bull Breeding Soundness Examination and Its Application in the Production Setting" in this issue.).

Although the practice is not recommended, some producers prefer to rent or lease bulls each year. This practice has the advantage of not having to maintain bulls during the nonbreeding season. However, it does pose a biosecurity risk if using a bull that was previously used in other herds. Bulls exposed to other herds may introduce reproductive diseases into the breeding herd. These bulls should be thoroughly tested before being introduced with cows. See Chapter 7—*Sexually Transmitted Diseases of Bulls* for testing recommendations.

## BULL-TO-COW RATIO (STOCKING RATE)

Common recommendations of bull-to-cow stocking ratio is one bull for every 25 or 30 cows.[2,5–8] This takes into account the potential that some bulls may become injured during the breeding season. Some studies have shown that fertile bulls can successfully breed 45 or more during a season.[16] Many bulls that pass a BSE can handle considerably more females in a breeding season than traditional recommendations.[17] Social ranking also impacts sexual activity and performance,[17,18] and dominance seems to be related to seniority.[3] Dominance may have a detrimental impact on reproductive efficiency if the dominant bull does not breed cows and prohibits subordinate bulls from breeding. Limiting factors to breeding potential of bulls include libido, breeding interference in multisire breeding groups and injury.[2,16,18] Inexperienced, yearling bulls should be exposed to fewer cows. A common recommendation for bulls with less than 2 years of age is one cow per month of age, assuming the bulls passed a BSE.[19]

## SUMMARY

When bulls are gathered from the breeding herd, it is a good time to sort and decide who needs to go and who is kept. After deciding who stays and who does not, it is important to decide how to care for the bulls in the off-season. Although bulls are tough and can be an aggravation to deal with, they are essential for reproductive efficiency of our cow herds. Proper care and maintenance in the off-season is crucial for optimal performance when the bull pen is called to get their job done. Ideally, the nonbreeding season management will result in bulls that are physically fit, fertile, and ready to perform their part for optimum reproductive efficiency in cow-calf operations.[5]

## DISCLOSURE

The Author has no COI to disclose. No funding was used in writing this manuscript.

## REFERENCES

1. USDA. Beef 2017, "beef cow-calf management practices in the United States, 2017, report 1. Fort Collins, CO: USDA–APHIS–VS–CEAH–NAHMS; 2020. #.782.0520.
2. Palmer CW. Management and Breeding Soundness of Mature Bulls. Vet Clin Food Anim 2016;32:479–95.
3. de Blockey MA. Observations on group mating of bulls at pasture. Appl Anim Ethol 1979;5:15–34.
4. Mueller M. Prevent bull fighting to mitigate injury in the offseason. Red Angus Magazine; 2023. p. 26–8.
5. King EH. Management of Breeding Bull Batteries. In: Hopper RM, editor. Bovine reproduction. 1st edition. Ames (IA): John Wiley and Sons, Inc.; 2015. p. 92–6.
6. R. Christmas. Management and Evaluation Considerations for Range Beef Bulls, in Topics in Bull Fertility by Chenowith P.J., 2001. Available at: https://www.ivis.org/library/topics-bull-fertility. (visited August 10, 2023).
7. K. H. Wilke, K. L. McCarthy, H. Greenwell. Breeding Bull Management: It's a Year-Round Commitment. UNL Nebguide G2332. March 2021 Available at: https://extensionpublications.unl.edu/assets/pdf/g2332.pdf (visited August 10, 2023)
8. Banwarth MR, DeAtley KL, Gifford CA, et al. Bull selection and management in extensive rangeland production systems of California: a producer survey. Trans Anim Sci 2022;6.
9. Barth AD, Waldner CL. Factors affecting breeding soundness classification of beef bulls examined at the Western College of Veterinary Medicine. Can Vet J 2002;43:274–84.
10. Capela L, Leites I, Romão R, et al. Impact of Heat Stress on Bovine Sperm Quality and Competence. Animals 2022;12(8):975.
11. Rowe MP, Powell JG, Kegley EB, et al. Effect of supplemental trace mineral source on bull semen quality. Prof Animal Sci 2014;30:68–73.
12. Clark BL, Duffy JH, Parsonson IM. Immunisation of bulls against trichomoniasis. Austr Vet Jour 1983;60:178–9.
13. Cobo ER, Corbeil LB, Gershwin LJ, et al. Preputial cellular and antibody responses of bulls vaccinated and/or challenged with Tritrichomonas foetus. Vaccine 2010;28:361–70.
14. Alling C, Rae DO, Ma X, et al. Systemic humoral immunity in beef bulls following therapeutic vaccination against Tritrichomonas foetus. Vet Parasit 2018;255:69–73.
15. Dohlman TM, Phillips PE, Madson DM, et al. Effects of label-dose permethrin administration in yearling beef cattle: I. Bull reproductive function and testicular histopathology. Therio 2016;85:1534–9.
16. Rupp GP, Ball L, Shoop MC, et al. Reproductive efficiency of bulls in natural service: effects of male to female ratio and single- vs multiple-sire breeding groups. JAVMA 1977;171:639–42.
17. Chenowith P. J., Bull Sex Drive and Reproductive Behavior, in Topics in Bull Fertility by Chenowith PJ. 2001. Available at: https://www.ivis.org/library/topics-bull-fertility. (visited August 10, 2023).
18. Fordyce G, Fitzpatrick LA, Cooper NJ, et al. Bull selection and use in northern Australia: 5. Social behaviour and management. Anim Reprod Sci 2002;71:81–99.
19. Wenzel J, Carson R, Wolfe D. Bull-to-cow ratios: practical formulae for estimating the number of bulls suggested for successful pasture breeding of female cattle. Clin Therio 2012;4:477–9.

# Genomics and Dairy Bull Fertility

Francisco Peñagaricano, PhD

## KEYWORDS

- Genomic prediction • Homozygosity • Major mutations • Sire conception rate

## KEY POINTS

- Genetic factors explain part of the differences observed in fertility among dairy bulls.
- There are mutations with large effects on bull fertility segregating in most dairy breeds.
- Genomic prediction of dairy bull fertility is feasible.
- Inbreeding and increased homozygosity negatively affect dairy bull fertility.

## REPRODUCTIVE EFFICIENCY IN DAIRY CATTLE

Reproductive efficiency is an extremely important economic trait in dairy cattle. Reproductive inefficiency results in increased calving intervals, increased involuntary culling rates, decreased milk production, and delayed genetic progress, among other problems.[1] Despite advances in the last 2 decades, mainly due to improvements in reproductive management, nutrition, and herd health, reproductive performance remains suboptimal in most dairy herds, resulting in significant economic losses for the dairy industry. For instance, the US Holstein breed averages 2.0 services per conception, around 114 days from calving to last breeding, 38 days from first to last breeding, 38% conception rate for first breeding, 35% conception rate for all breedings, and a calving interval of almost 400 days.[2] Therefore, there is a clear need for the scientific community and the dairy industry to develop new strategies and tools to improve dairy cattle reproductive performance.

## DAIRY BULL FERTILITY

Reproduction is a complex process that involves many consecutive events, including gametogenesis, fertilization, and early embryo development, that should be accomplished in a well-orchestrated manner to achieve a successful pregnancy. Although both parents affect the reproductive success,[3] much of the research on dairy cattle has focused on cow fertility, while the potential contributions of the bull have been largely ignored. This seems to be contradictory considering that semen from one bull is used to inseminate hundreds of cows, and thus, one subfertile bull would

Department of Animal and Dairy Sciences, University of Wisconsin-Madison
*E-mail address:* fpenagarican@wisc.edu

Vet Clin Food Anim 40 (2024) 185–190
https://doi.org/10.1016/j.cvfa.2023.08.005
0749-0720/24/© 2023 Elsevier Inc. All rights reserved.

have a larger effect on the overall herd fertility than a single cow with fertility problems. In fact, several reports have shown that a significant percentage of reproductive failure is attributable to bull subfertility.[4,5] There is growing evidence that paternal factors directly contribute to pregnancy success. Indeed, recent studies have shown that the reduced ability of low-fertility bulls to establish pregnancy is multifactorial, including sperm fertilizing ability, preimplantation embryonic development, and placenta and embryo development after conceptus elongation and pregnancy recognition.[6,7] Therefore, the fertility of service sires should not be overlooked in breeding schemes aimed at improving the reproductive performance of dairy cattle.

## EVALUATING DAIRY BULL FERTILITY

Dairy bull fertility has been traditionally evaluated in the laboratory based on semen analysis. This approach uses conventional laboratory methods, which measures semen production traits, such as volume and sperm concentration, and semen quality traits, such as motility and percentage of abnormal sperm.[8] Unfortunately, these sperm quality traits explain only part of the differences observed in fertility among dairy sires, and significant fertility differences exist among bulls producing spermatozoa with normal motility, morphology, and count.[9] Alternatively, bull fertility can be directly evaluated using cow field records. One could argue that the true fertility of a bull should be measured in the field, and the semen traits measured in the laboratory should be considered as indicator traits. Indeed, United States and Australia have developed national evaluations of dairy bull fertility using confirmed pregnancy records and nonreturn to service records, respectively. It should be noted that most national evaluations for fertility are limited to female fertility traits, and evaluations for bull fertility traits are commonly undertaken by individual breeding organizations and usually not made public.[10]

## SIRE CONCEPTION RATE

Since 2008, US dairy farmers have access to a national phenotypic evaluation of service sire fertility called sire conception rate (SCR). This bull fertility evaluation is exclusively based on cow field data. The current evaluation model includes both factors related to the service sire under evaluation, including age of the bull and artificial insemination (AI) organization, and factors (nuisance variables) associated with the cow that receives the unit of semen, including herd-year-season, cow age, parity, and milk yield. The trait SCR is defined as the expected difference in conception rate of a given bull compared with the mean of all other evaluated bulls; in other words, a bull with an SCR value of +5.0% is expected to achieve a conception rate of 36% in a herd that normally averages 31% and uses average SCR bulls. Contrary to evaluations for other traits such as milk production or cow fertility, SCR is designed as a phenotypic rather than a genetic evaluation because the published estimates include not only genetic but also nongenetic effects. Currently, there are about 15,800 Holstein bulls and 2050 Jersey bulls with official SCR evaluations. Interestingly, there is a remarkable variation in SCR both in Holsteins and in Jerseys; indeed, there are more than 15 points (15% conception rate difference) between the 2 extremes, that is, between high-fertility and low-fertility bulls.

## GENETIC FACTORS AFFECT DAIRY BULL FERTILITY

Two pioneer genomics studies in US Holstein[11] and US Jersey[12] revealed that (1) genetic factors do explain part of the variation in SCR; (2) most of the significant genomic regions are breed-specific, and this may be due to multiple reasons, such as different causal mutations, differences in linkage disequilibrium pattern, or simply false-positive/false-negative results; and (3) most of the significant gene-sets are common to both breeds, and this provides further evidence that pathways rather than single genes are the primary target of selection. A recent study in Italian Brown Swiss cattle[13] confirmed these initial findings: part of the variation in SCR is explained by genetic factors, most of the significant regions are breed-specific, and there are numerous gene-sets, including cell migration, cell–cell interaction, GTPase activity, and immune function that affect bull fertility across different dairy breeds.

## MAJOR MUTATIONS AFFECTING DAIRY BULL FERTILITY

Complex phenotypes tend to be modulated by many genes, all of them with small effects. However, in the case of dairy bull fertility, recent studies have revealed major mutations affecting SCR in different dairy breeds. In Holsteins, there are 5 genomic regions, located on bovine chromosome (BTA) 8 (72.2 Mb), BTA 9 (43.7 Mb), BTA 13 (60.2 Mb), BTA 17 (63.3 Mb), and BTA 27 (34.7 Mb), which show very significant effects on bull fertility.[14,15] Each of these regions explains about 5% to 8% of the observed differences in conception rate between Holstein bulls. The targeted sequencing of these 5 regions identified a set of deleterious mutations, including missense and frameshift variants.[16] Most of these mutations are located on genes exclusively or highly expressed in testis. In Jerseys, there are 2 genomic regions, located on BTA 11 (2.6 Mb) and BTA 25 (19.1 Mb), which show very significant effects on SCR.[12] Each of these regions explains about 4% to 6% of the observed differences in fertility between Jersey bulls and harbors some strong candidate genes, such as *FER1L5*, *CNNM4*, and *DNAH3*, with known roles in sperm biology. In Brown Swiss, several independent studies have identified one genomic region on BTA 6 (57.6 Mb) that negatively influences numerous bull fertility traits, including sperm motility, sperm abnormalities, insemination success, and SCR.[13,17,18] This region harbors gene *WDR19*, which is a constituent of the intraflagellar transport complex that is essential for the physiologic function of motile cilia and flagella, including sperm motility.[19] Overall, although bull fertility is undoubtedly a complex trait modulated by many genes, there are some mutations with large effect segregating in different dairy cattle populations. These major mutations could be used to screen and detect subfertile bull calves.

## GENOMIC PREDICTION OF DAIRY BULL FERTILITY

The advent of genomic prediction in the last decade has transformed dairy cattle breeding, enabling more rapid genetic progress, particularly for low heritable traits while facilitating the selection for novel traits. Interestingly, several studies have shown that the genomic prediction of service sire fertility is feasible. These studies have reported prediction accuracies up to 0.65 in US Holstein[20] and around 0.60 in US Jersey.[21] Just as reference, health traits, such as ketosis and metritis, have accuracies around 0.55 to 0.60, and feed efficiency, one of the latest traits included in the US national genetic evaluation, has prediction accuracies around 0.30. Further research showed that the use of biological information, such as markers with large effect or functional data, or the inclusion of sex chromosome markers, yields even better predictions of dairy bull fertility.[15,22] Given that bull fertility is time-consuming, difficult to measure, and most databases are relatively small, Rezende and collaborators evaluated the use of an across-country reference population combining records from the United States and Australia to predict service sire fertility in Jersey cattle.[23] They corroborated that genomic prediction of dairy bull fertility is feasible, and they suggested that the use of an across-country reference population would be beneficial when local populations are small and genetically diverse. Overall, genomic prediction of bull fertility is feasible in dairy cattle. Note that bull fertility records, such SCR records, are available only after the bulls are in the market, and hence, early genomic predictions can help the dairy industry make accurate genome-guided selection decisions, such as early culling of predicted subfertile bull calves.

## INBREEDING, HOMOZYGOSITY, AND DAIRY BULL FERTILITY

Dairy cattle breeding programs currently face the challenge of achieving rapid genetic progress while maintaining adequate genetic diversity and low inbreeding levels. Inbreeding, the mating of related individuals, cannot be avoided in populations of limited size but it is especially exacerbated in dairy cattle due to intense selection and heavy use of artificial insemination. The increase in inbreeding tends to impact performance, especially fitness-related traits, such as fertility. Traditionally, inbreeding has been monitored using pedigree information, or more recently, genomic data. Alternatively, inbreeding can be quantified using runs of homozygosity, defined as runs of consecutive homozygous genotypes observed in an individual's chromosome. Notably, genomic studies conducted in both Holstein and Brown Swiss have reported negative associations between bull fertility, measured as SCR, and the amount of homozygosity, calculated as the sum of runs of homozygosity.[24,25] Both studies showed that low-fertility bulls have significantly higher levels of homozygosity than high-fertility bulls. In addition, both studies found that those homozygote regions significantly enriched in low-fertility bulls harbor many genes closely related to sperm biology and male fertility, including genes exclusively or highly expressed in testis. Overall, these studies suggest that inbreeding and the increase in homozygosity, that is, the loss of genetic diversity, have a negative impact on dairy bull fertility.

## OTHER OMICS TECHNOLOGIES

There are other biological markers, besides genetic variants, that could be used to identify low-fertility/high-fertility bulls. In fact, several transcriptomic, proteomic, and metabolomic studies have discovered numerous differences between the spermatozoa of high-fertility versus low-fertility bulls.[26–28] Gross and collaborators found a total of 65 RNAs to be differentially expressed between 2 to 4 cell bovine embryos derived from high-fertility and low-fertility dairy bulls.[29] As a proof of principle, these researchers knocked down one differentially expressed RNA (ATXN2L), which led to a 23% increase in blastocyst development. These findings provide evidence that paternally contributed RNAs are important for bovine embryo development, and these RNAs could be used as biomarkers to predict bull fertility. DNA methylation is another biomarker that could be used to predict dairy bull fertility. Indeed, several studies have identified DNA methylation differences between the spermatozoa of high-fertility versus low-fertility bulls.[30–32] Interestingly, many of these differentially methylated cytosines are in genes related to sperm biology and early embryonic development. Overall, the identification of biomarkers for bull fertility could assist farmers, breeders, and AI companies in making accurate management and selection decisions, such as using or marketing semen from high-fertility bulls or early culling of predicted subfertile bull calves.[33]

## SUMMARY

There is a remarkable variation in SCR among dairy bulls, with more than 10% conception rate difference between high-fertility and low-fertility bulls. Interestingly, part of this variation is explained by genetic factors. Although dairy bull fertility is undoubtedly a complex trait modulated by many genes, several studies have shown that there are some major mutations segregating in most dairy breeds. In fact, each of these major mutations explains about 4% to 8% of the observed differences in conception rate between bulls. Research has also shown that genomic prediction of dairy bull fertility is feasible. Given that bull fertility records are available only after the bulls are in the market, early genomic predictions could be used to make accurate selection and management decisions, such as early culling of predicted subfertile bull calves. Inbreeding tends to affect performance, especially fitness-related traits, and recent studies have shown that inbreeding and the increase in homozygosity negatively affect dairy bull fertility. Overall, dairy bull fertility is influenced by genetic factors, and hence, it could be managed and improved by genetic means.

## DISCLOSURE

The author has not stated any conflicts of interest.

## REFERENCES

1. Weigel KA. Prospects for improving reproductive performance through genetic selection. Anim Reprod Sci 2006;96(3–4):323–30.
2. Norman HD, Guinan FL, Megonigal JH, Durr JW. Reproductive status of cows in Dairy Herd Improvement programs and bred using artificial insemination. 2020. Available at: https://queries.uscdcb.com/publish/dhi/current/reproall.html.
3. Kropp J, Peñagaricano F, Salih SM, et al. Invited review: Genetic contributions underlying the development of preimplantation bovine embryos. J Dairy Sci 2014; 97(3):1187–201.
4. Nagamine Y, Sasaki O. Effect of environmental factors on fertility of Holstein-Friesian cattle in Japan. Livest Sci 2008;115(1):89–93.
5. Amann RP, DeJarnette JM. Impact of genomic selection of AI dairy sires on their likely utilization and methods to estimate fertility: A paradigm shift. Theriogenology 2012;77(5):795–817.
6. Ortega MS, Moraes JGN, Patterson DJ, et al. Influences of sire conception rate on pregnancy establishment in dairy cattle. Biol Reprod 2018;99(6):1244–54.
7. Immler S. The sperm factor: paternal impact beyond genes. Heredity 2018; 121(3):239–47.
8. DeJarnette JM, Marshall CE, Lenz RW, et al. Sustaining the fertility of artificially inseminated dairy cattle: the role of the artificial insemination industry. J Dairy Sci 2004;87(Supplement):E93–104.
9. Parkinson TJ. Evaluation of fertility and infertility in natural service bulls. Vet J 2004;168(3):215–29.
10. Berry DP, Evans RD, Mc Parland S. Evaluation of bull fertility in dairy and beef cattle using cow field data. Theriogenology 2011;75(1):172–81.
11. Han Y, Peñagaricano F. Unravelling the genomic architecture of bull fertility in Holstein cattle. BMC Genet 2016;17(1):143.
12. Rezende FM, Dietsch GO, Peñagaricano F. Genetic dissection of bull fertility in US Jersey dairy cattle. Anim Genet 2018;49(5):393–402.
13. Pacheco HA, Rossoni A, Cecchinato A, et al. Deciphering the genetic basis of male fertility in Italian Brown Swiss dairy cattle. Sci Rep 2022;12(1):10575.
14. Nicolini P, Amorin R, Han Y, et al. Whole-genome scan reveals significant non-additive effects for sire conception rate in Holstein cattle. BMC Genet 2018; 19(1):14.

15. Nani JP, Rezende FM, Peñagaricano F. Predicting male fertility in dairy cattle using markers with large effect and functional annotation data. BMC Genom 2019; 20(1):258.

16. Abdollahi-Arpanahi R, Pacheco HA, Peñagaricano F. Targeted sequencing reveals candidate causal variants for dairy bull subfertility. Anim Genet 2021; 52(4):509–13.

17. Hiltpold M, Niu G, Kadri NK, et al. Activation of cryptic splicing in bovine WDR19 is associated with reduced semen quality and male fertility. PLoS Genet 2020; 16(5):e1008804.

18. Mapel XM, Hiltpold M, Kadri NK, et al. Bull fertility and semen quality are not correlated with dairy and production traits in Brown Swiss cattle. JDS Communications 2022;3(2):120–5.

19. Ni X, Wang J, Lv M, et al. A novel homozygous mutation in WDR19 induces disorganization of microtubules in sperm flagella and nonsyndromic asthenoteratospermia. J Assist Reprod Genet 2020;37(6):1431–9.

20. Abdollahi-Arpanahi R, Morota G, Peñagaricano F. Predicting bull fertility using genomic data and biological information. J Dairy Sci 2017;100(12):9656–66.

21. Rezende FM, Nani JP, Peñagaricano F. Genomic prediction of bull fertility in US Jersey dairy cattle. J Dairy Sci 2019;102(4):3230–40.

22. Pacheco HA, Rezende FM, Peñagaricano F. Gene mapping and genomic prediction of bull fertility using sex chromosome markers. J Dairy Sci 2020;103(4): 3304–11.

23. Rezende FM, Haile-Mariam M, Pryce JE, et al. Across-country genomic prediction of bull fertility in Jersey dairy cattle. J Dairy Sci 2020;103(12):11618–27.

24. Nani JP, Peñagaricano F. Whole-genome homozygosity mapping reveals candidate regions affecting bull fertility in US Holstein cattle. BMC Genom 2020; 21(1):338.

25. Pacheco HA, Rossoni A, Cecchinato A, et al. Identification of runs of homozygosity associated with male fertility in Brown Swiss cattle. Front Genet 2023;14: 1227310.

26. Prakash MA, Kumaresan A, Ebenezer Samuel King JP, et al. Comparative Transcriptomic Analysis of Spermatozoa From High- and Low-Fertile Crossbred Bulls: Implications for Fertility Prediction. Front Cell Dev Biol 2021;9:647717.

27. Dasgupta M, Kumaresan A, Saraf KK, et al. Deep Metabolomic Profiling Reveals Alterations in Fatty Acid Synthesis and Ketone Body Degradations in Spermatozoa and Seminal Plasma of Astheno-Oligozoospermic Bulls. Front Vet Sci 2021;8: 755560.

28. Kaya A, Dogan S, Vargovic P, et al. Sperm proteins ODF2 and PAWP as markers of fertility in breeding bulls. Cell Tissue Res 2022;387(1):159–71.

29. Gross N, Strillacci MG, Peñagaricano F, et al. Characterization and functional roles of paternal RNAs in 2-4 cell bovine embryos. Sci Rep 2019;9(1):20347.

30. Gross N, Peñagaricano F, Khatib H. Integration of whole-genome DNA methylation data with RNA sequencing data to identify markers for bull fertility. Anim Genet 2020;51(4):502–10.

31. Zhang Y, Bruna de Lima C, Labrecque R, et al. Whole-genome DNA methylation analysis of the sperm in relation to bull fertility. Reproduction 2023;165(5):557–68.

32. Štiavnická M, Chaulot-Talmon A, Perrier JP, et al. Sperm DNA methylation patterns at discrete CpGs and genes involved in embryonic development are related to bull fertility. BMC Genom 2022;23(1):379.

33. Klein EK, Swegen A, Gunn AJ, et al. The future of assessing bull fertility: Can the 'omics fields identify useable biomarkers? Biol Reprod 2022;106(5):854–64.

# Moving?

## Make sure your subscription moves with you!

To notify us of your new address, find your **Clinics Account Number** (located on your mailing label above your name), and contact customer service at:

**Email: journalscustomerservice-usa@elsevier.com**

**800-654-2452** (subscribers in the U.S. & Canada)
**314-447-8871** (subscribers outside of the U.S. & Canada)

**Fax number: 314-447-8029**

**Elsevier Health Sciences Division**
**Subscription Customer Service**
**3251 Riverport Lane**
**Maryland Heights, MO 63043**

*To ensure uninterrupted delivery of your subscription, please notify us at least 4 weeks in advance of move.

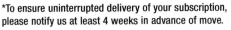